TABLE OF CONTENTS

INTRODUCTION

The ketogenic diet can be a terribly low-carbohydrate diet, high in fat, and have several similarities to the Atkins diet and the low-sugar diet.

This diet involves a drastic reduction in sugar intake and replacing it with carbohydrates, which I believe is an extremely metabolic state known as ketonemia.

When this happens, your body is unlikely to be economical in converting fat into energy. It also converts fats into ketones in the liver, which can provide energy to the brain.

The ketogenic diet has been gaining quality for a number of years for its various benefits, as well as weight loss and improved health. Unlike various fashionable diets, the "keto" is not a cult and should remain. Several studies have indeed demonstrated the benefits of the ketogenic diet in the context of polygenic disorder, metabolic syndrome, epilepsy, and Alzheimer's disease, among others.

Many keto clinics and diet specialists around the world currently offer the services of the Keto Consultation. Their goal is to help people gain and maintain a healthy weight and improve their polygenic disorder and various metabolic problems through a complete nutritional approach, without supplements or prepackaged meals. Dr. Registered dietitians, Elyssa Elman, and Lauren Richer have been serving patients for years to reduce and restore their health.

WHAT IS THE KETOGENIC DIET?

The ketogenic diet can be low carbohydrate, high fat, and moderate in the super molecule diet. By drastically reducing the intake of saccharide and providing the body with sufficient fat, the body goes from burning sugar to victim fat as fuel. This can be referred to as the biological process of acetonemia. Once this happens, the body effectively burns fat and restores its energy. This diet will bring about significant improvements in the levels of aldohexose and internal secretion, as well as several useful facet effects such as mental clarity, improved energy levels, and increased concentration.

What is the biological process of ketosis? Is it constant like ketoacidosis?

Ketosis can be a natural metabolic state in which fats provide fuel for the body and also for the brain. Once the body uses fat as a fuel, it breaks it down, and also, the by-product of this method produces ketones. In the case of acetonemia, it is usually necessary to consume only forty g of internet carbohydrates per day and even up to only twenty g of carbohydrates per day. Ketoacidosis, on the other hand, can be a deadly disease related to polygenic disease, caused by terribly high levels of ketones and sugar in the blood. This condition causes various symptoms and even death. A low carbohydrate diet causes acetonemia, while poor treatment of the polygenic disease is the main trigger for diabetic acidosis.

Types of Keto Diet

There are different forms of the ketogenic diet as follows: The standard diet is incredibly low in carbohydrates, moderate in a macromolecule, and high in fat.

It always contains 75% fat, 20% macromolecule, and only 5% carbohydrates. The cyclic keto diet contains high peri-molecular periods, such as five ketogenic days followed by two carbohydrate-rich days. Another focused keto diet has carbohydrates around workouts.

High macromolecule ketogenic diet: It is a kind of everyday ketogenic diet, but contains extra protein. The quantitative relationship is usually 60% fat, 35% macromolecule, and 5% supermolecule. Know that only every day and highly macromolecular ketogenic diets are studied extensively.

Cyclical or targeted ketogenic diets are additional advanced strategies, mainly used by bodybuilders or athletes. The information in this article applies mainly to the quality ketogenic diet (SKD).

Ketogenic diets will lead to massive reductions in glucose levels and internal secretion. This, in addition, is the increase of the ketones, has a number of health edges. Ketogenic diets can help you lose weight:
A ketogenic diet is good thanks to slim and reduces the risk factors for disease.   In fact, telling analysis is that the ketogenic diet is the superior way of guiding the diet by several. In addition, this diet is, therefore, satisfying that you simply lose weight without adding up calories or following the food consumed.
One study found that individuals on a ketogenic diet lost twice as much weight a few times than those on a calorie-restricted diet. Lipid and cholesterol levels improved at the same time. There are many reasons why the ketogenic diet is healthier than a diet. One is an increased intake of supermolecules that offers different edges.
Increasing ketones, lowering blood glucose levels, and increasing sensitivity to hypoglycemic agents can also play a key role.

Why consume a lot of fat? Is it dangerous?

 When we limit saccharin intake, fat becomes our primary energy supplier. Dietary fats have different functions in the body, apart from energy, which serves as the North American nation absorb vitamins, regulate inflammation and immunity, saturation, and repairs just what to call. Fat is in every animal (meat, fish, eggs) and vegetable sources (avocado, oil, olives). Although fat has gotten a bad name over the years, studies have found no link between saturated fat and cardiomyopathy. It is necessary to vary your fat sources. All fats are not created equal; why is their fat to avoid, then there are fats that are smart for your health.
 With a ketogenic diet, we tend to use a few tablespoons of fat per meal. This is tasty and can be a great way to add flavor to a meal!
I usually browse that the ketogenic diet helps treat the metabolic syndrome; however, what is it?
Metabolic syndrome can increase a cluster of disorders that commonly occur and the risk of cardiomyopathy, stroke, and polygenic disorders. One in five people has an identification of the metabolic syndrome. It is diagnosed once a person has at least 3 of the following conditions:

- Hypertension
- High blood glucose

- High triglycerides
- Low cholesterol
- High waist

I am disaccharide intolerant; can I still follow this type of diet?
Following a ketogenic diet does not have the consumption of dairy farm products. Dairy farm product is a fair supply of fat and macromolecule, just like Ca, vitamin D, and phosphorus. However, it is not essential during this diet. There are several alternatives to the dairy product s and a range of ketogenic recipes that do not embody dairy to do while still delicious.

I travel a lot and have to eat a lot, is that a problem?

The ketogenic diet would be an approach to life, and could simply work into your busy schedule, whether it be consumption, travel, or just going out.
It is very easy to crumble the building during this program. A Keto Diet Authority will teach you what you want to understand to make the right selections after eating out and can provide you with a guide to make you feel cozy where you are.

I take medicines, is that diet safe for me?

A specialized custom keto diet program is managed by a team of qualified professionals, as well as doctors. If changes are needed, one of the specialists/doctors can guide you in creating a positive result by taking the right doses.
Many patients do not follow a program like this to achieve treatment for their polygenic disorder and, as a result, will cut back or stop taking most, if not all, of their medications, as well as hypoglycemic agents and looking for healthy low carb diet ideas?
Discover this simple, delicious, and friendly recipe:

Pizza Keto

Ingredients

- The rind: ½ cup of grated cheese
- ¾ cup of almond flour
- 2 tablespoons. cheese
- 1 egg
- garlic salt
- Topping options:
- tomato sauce
- Pesto
- Cheese
- Fresh herbs
- Vegetables
- olives
- Pepperoni
- Sausage

- Chicken.

DIRECTION:

1. Place the cheese and cheese in a medium microwave bowl.
2. Heat for a minute, stir, and microwave for another thirty seconds.
3. Stir in the egg and, consequently, the almond flour.
4. Wet your hands and unfold the dough on baking paper.
5. Drill rows of holes in the dough to avoid air bubbles.
6. Sprinkle with sea salt.
7. Put in the kitchen appliance at physicist 425 degrees.
8. After eight minutes, check the dough and drill additional holes if necessary.
9. Cook for another 12 to 14 minutes or until the dough is golden brown.
10. Add your favorite toppings according to your style.

WHO SHOULD KETO DIET?

A keto diet is high in fat and low in carbohydrates—for example, egg, butter, sugar-free drinks, etc. A ketogenic diet could basically be considered a low carb diet, and the concept is a way to get extra energy from macromolecule and fat and much less from carbohydrates. You chop back most with the carbohydrates that are easy to digest, such as sugar, soft drinks, pastries, and vitality. If you eat a lot of fifty grams of carbohydrates every day, your body will run out of gasoline (blood sugar) within the finish and can use it quickly. This sometimes takes 3 to 4 days. Then you start interrupting macromolecules and fats for strength, which may make you less. This is often called acetonemia. It is vital to note that the ketogenic weight-reduction could be a temporary food plan. This often focuses on weight loss rather than pursuing health benefits. Individuals usually use a ketogenic diet to reduce. Hof added it is going to help manage positive scientific conditions, such as brain disease, too. It can also be people with a heart condition, positive brain diseases, and disorders even easier, but there are additional studies in those fields required.

Talk to your health professional first to see if it is safe so you can try a ketogenic diet plan, especially after you have some type of polygenic condition. A ketogenic nutrition system can also help you lose extra weight within the primary three to six months than some completely different diets. As a result, more calories are needed to convert fat into strength than to convert carbohydrates into strength. It is also viable that a high-fat diet satisfies you extra; therefore, you eat less, but that has not been proven, however. Insulin can be a separation that we tend to your body or use sugar as a fuel store. Ketogenic diets help you burn this gas quickly, so you don't want to avoid wasting it. This fashion that your body wants - and makes - much less internal secretion. In addition, those lower values can help protect you against a number of cancers or perhaps slow the emergence of cancer cells.

However, this requires additional analysis. It seems strange that a weight loss program that the question at greater fats will increase "good" cholesterol and lower "bad" LDL cholesterol; however, ketogenic diets are only linked to that. It will ensure that the decrease in internal secretions resulting from these diets will prevent your body from creating higher cholesterol. That way, you're less likely to grand total high power per unit area, arteriosclerosis, have heart disease, coronary heart disease, and alternative. However, it is not clear, ever, how long those effects last. Carbohydrates are linked to the power source skin condition, so cutting on them can, moreover, facilitate. And also, it is due to the internal secretion that will trigger a ketogenic consumption plan that can also facilitate stop breakouts. (Insulin will use your body to create alternative hormones that cause bursts.) Still, additional analysis is needed to make a precise decision; however, tons of impact, if any, the consumption plan actually has on pimples. A ketogenic diet can facilitate endurance athletes - runners and cyclists, for example - once they have trained. Over time, it helps your muscle-to-fat magnitude relationship and increases the number eight that your body is in an extraordinary position to use once in exercise. But while it would facilitate employment, it should not additionally work as different diets for peak performance.

The extra common ones are usually not serious: you would probably have constipation, delicate low glucose, or symptoms. Abundantly less often, low-carb diets can cause urinary tract stones or high acid levels in your body (acidosis). Various aspect effects may include the "keto respiratory disease," which may include headache, weakness and irritability; dangerous breath; and fatigue.

When your body burns its stored fat, it should strain your kidneys. And starting a healthy ketogenic diet - or going back to a normal diet later - is also tricky if you're suffering from health problems you're likely to have, such as polygenic disorder, cardiopathy, or high strength per unit space. If you have any of these conditions, make dietary changes slowly and only under the direction of your doctor. Switching to a ketogenic diet can seem overwhelming, but it doesn't have to be robust.

Your focus should be forced to reduce carbohydrates while increasing the amount of fat and organic compounds in meals and snacks. To achieve and maintain a very high state of ketosis, carbohydrates must be limited.

While positive people can only follow ketosis through intake; however, twenty grams of carbohydrates per day, others might even be sure with much higher carbohydrate intake. In general, the lower your sugar intake, the less complicated it is to achieve and maintain ketosis. This is why reaching out for keto-friendly foods and avoiding things loaded in carbohydrates is the easiest to initiate a ketogenic diet successfully.

The keto diet needs the body to fully believe in fat for energy, rather than the same old carbohydrates (see Carbohydrates vs. Fat for Fuel below). Once carbohydrate intake is incredibly low, ketones - products of fat breakdown in the liver - should fuel the body.

There is no international definition of the ketogenic diet. In other words, there is no custom on how to consume a few grams of saccharide, fat, or supermolecule after the diet.

Most dietary analyzes have seen a saccharide intake between twenty-five and fifty grams per day, such as 2 medium apples or a cup of cooked rice. This extreme saccharide reduction is incredibly difficult to take care of in the long term and does not make it possible to meet the suggested amount of fruits, vegetables, and whole-grain portions suggested for a healthy diet. In accordance with the Diet Guides for Americans, carbohydrates should be up to forty-five to sixty pc daily calories, or one hundred and thirty grams/day, for many people to eat a diet and acquire the necessary nutrients.

For patients with encephalopathy, ketogenic diets are administered in an extraordinarily clinical setting, and they need a team of dieticians and doctors to confirm that patients are getting the right amount of nutrients every day - and they are still extremely tiring to follow.

In addition to the lower carbohydrate intake, another important part of the diet is the extraordinarily high intake of dietary fat. Overpowering most of the calories from fat and severely limiting saccharide keeps the body in an extraordinary state of ketonemia (completely dependent on ketones for energy).

Short-term weight loss can occur naturally, largely due to the water weight you lose. Your body can eat its animal starch reserves (regular energy reserves due to the breakdown of saccharides) and also the water it retains. While many people decrease quickly, it is water weight, not really weight loss. In most cases, the burden can come when the diet again contains a higher proportion of carbohydrates. For that reason, the ketogenic diet is unlikely to facilitate long-term weight loss.

The keto diet is not for everyone. Certainly, if you have glucose problems or a history of heart disease, you should not do that diet while not under a doctor's supervision. However, if you're healthy and trying to find a jump start for weight loss, the keto diet might just be the chance you're trying to find. This diet is not acceptable for people with a stage of polygenic disease, uropathy or pre-existing liver, exocrine gland, or excretory organ problems or conditions. Some rare conditions, such as hereditary disease and alternative conditions, can complicate and discomfort the exocrine system, liver, or kidneys.

This diet is not acceptable under any circumstances if you currently have glucose problems such as hypoglycemia or sorting a polygenic disease. It may or may not be acceptable if you have two types of polygenic diseases and are taking diabetes drugs, and may need physician supervision. This diet may not be acceptable or safe for people who are pregnant, breastfeeding, or have a physiological condition with the polygenic disease.

This diet may not be acceptable for the first degree suffering from or recovering from a disorder.

HAVE YOU PLANNED TO YOUR FAVORITE DIET FOR the YEAR 2020 TO CHOOSE

In the field of dieting, there is no shortage of recommendations. Magazines, books, and websites all promise that you will lose all the burden you would want to lose permanently, operating diets that eliminate fat or carbohydrates, or people who recommend superfoods or special supplements.

But do you understand, with so many conflicting choices, that this approach might work for you? Here are some suggestions for selecting a weight loss program. Consult your doctor before starting a weight loss program. Your doctor will assess your medical problems and medications that may have an effect on your weight and provide you with a program for you. And you will discuss a way to exercise safely, especially if you have physical or medical challenges or pain from daily tasks.

Tell your doctor about your previous weight loss attempts. Be open about fashion diets that interest you. Your doctor may be ready to refer you to weight loss support teams or refer you to a registered specialist. There is no one to take care of everyone. However, if you think about your weight loss preferences, fashion, and goals, you will likely notice a concept that you can adapt to your liking.

Benefits of the keto diet

1. Help lose weight

It takes a lot of work to convert energy than to convert carbohydrates into energy. As a result, a ketogenic diet will accelerate weight loss.

And since the diet is high in a macromolecule, it doesn't leave you hungry like different diets. In a meta-analysis of thirteen completely different irregularly controlled studies, five outcomes revealed vital weight loss from the ketogenic diet.

2. Reduces skin condition

There are various causes of skin conditions, and one is also associated with diet and blood glucose. Ingestion of a diet high in processed and refined carbohydrates will change the intestinal bacteria, and many cause dramatic fluctuations in blood glucose, each of which can affect the health of the skin. Therefore, by reducing carbohydrate intake, it is no surprise that a ketogenic diet can reduce some cases of skin condition.

3. It can reduce the risk of cancer.

Ketogenic has proven to be a good deal on how it will prevent or perhaps treat certain cancers. A study showed that the ketogenic diet is also an acceptable complementary treatment for therapy and radiation in people with cancer. It may be because it causes much aerobic stress in cancer cells than in traditional cells.
Other theories suggest that as a result of the ketogenic diet lowers high blood glucose, and it may reduce the complications of hypoglycemic agents, which may be related to some cancers.

4. Improves heart health

When the ketogenic diet is followed in a healthy way (which considers avocados a healthy fat rather than pork rind), there is some evidence that the diet will improve heart health by reducing cholesterin. A study showed that high density ("good") cholesterin lipoprotein is significantly hyperbolic in those on the keto diet. The LDL ("bad") cholesterin decreased significantly.

5. can protect the functioning of the brain

More research is needed on the keto diet and, therefore, the brain. Some studies suggest that the keto diet offers neuroprotective benefits. These can treat or facilitate preventable conditions such as Parkinson's, Alzheimer's, and various disorders. Researchers found that the generation of young people that a ketogenic diet followed, alertness, and functioning of psychological functions had improved.

6. undoubtedly reduces attacks

The mix of fat, protein, and carbohydrates is thought to change the way the body uses energy, leading to symptoms. The symptom is Associate in a Nursing increased level of organic compound bodies in the blood.

Ketosis will result in a reduction in seizures in people with brain disease. The jury remains informed, how effective this is, although it seems best to have children. UN agency has focal attacks.

7. **Improves health in ladies with PCOS**

Polycystic female internal reproductive organ syndrome (PCOS) is an endocrine condition that causes enlarged ovaries with cysts. A carbohydrate-rich diet has a negative effect on people with PCOS.

There are not several clinical studies on the ketogenic diet and PCOS. A pilot study involving five ladies over a 24-week period found that the ketogenic diet:

- increased weight loss
- secretion balance helped
- improved ratios of gonadotropic hormone (LH) / follicle-stimulating hormone (FSH)
- improved hypoglycemic rapidly
- More analysis is needed.

Risks and complications

The ketogenic diet can have health benefits, as well as rapid weight loss. However, it is imperative to note that staying on the ketogenic diet for a long time has adverse effects on your health.

These include the risk of severe weight loss or muscle degeneration   (for long-term use). In several cases, the direct facet effects of the diet can be:

- constipation
- slowness
- low blood glucose

These symptoms are especially common at the beginning of the diet as your body adapts. The main and most popular energy supply for your brain and body comes from aldohexose. As a result, a powerful carbohydrate elimination is usually not a property technique to achieve optimal optimism.

Take any powerful change in your diet has potential health effects. As a result, you should constantly consult your doctor or dietitian before starting a replacement diet. If you are fascinated with starting the keto diet, you should be careful to investigate with your doctor whether you have a polygenic condition, hypoglycemia, or cardiovascular disease.

Since you don't want your body to show symptoms for too long, you will want to discuss several nutritional choices for an Associate in a nurse for a longer period of time. The ketogenic diet eliminates and refines carbohydrates in a much better form, but not all carbohydrates are created equal. Several health benefits come from a diet with a range of nutrient-rich, fibrous carbohydrates, fruits, vegetables, lean proteins, and healthy fats.

There is a known facet effect of the keto diet, some of which can be unpleasant. Some facet effects of the keto diet are absolutely present, although others only occur if the diet is poorly maintained.

The keto diet should not lead to some negative facet effects. But anyone considering long-term diet should be particularly careful.

The keto diet is usually referred to as an obese diet. Make no mistake: it is. However, not like alternative, stylish diets, the keto diet is exclusive in that it really pushes the body to vary degrees, a natural metabolic state called ketonemia. Once this happens, you can reliably expect many negative facet effects, especially those that go along with the 'keto respiratory disorder.' However, alternative facet effects are emerging, and only people are poorly performing the keto diet, generally by not eating a balanced, nutrient-rich food as part of a low-fat, low-carb diet. What can happen after you've taken common sources of fiber from your diet? Constipation. As a result, ketogenic eaters lack the benefits of a high-fiber diet, such as regular laxation and support of the microbiome. The microbiome has been involved in everything from immune performance to mental state. "

However, the keto diet is not g e t lead to fiber shortage: avocados, flax seeds, almonds, pecans, and chia seeds will all provide fiber, while still taking into account ketonemia - ever consumed in the right amounts.

Any diet that forbids you from feeding many fruits, vegetables, and alternative foods are absolute to put you at risk for food and mineral deficiencies, which is why several doctors only recommend following the short-term keto diet. With the keto diet, your body begins to lose fat, water, and animal starch, and when it does, you lose important electrolytes, such as Na, metal, and metal. If you are running low on these electrolytes, you may experience headaches or extreme fatigue. These losses are most pronounced during the first few weeks of entering ketonemia.

Thus, if you are striving to start the keto diet, it is best to plan ahead to get certain healthy amounts of these electrolytes - and alternative vitamins and minerals - either through supplements or a carefully designed design. One of the main direct facet effects of the keto diet is that the "keto respiratory disorder" is a collection of symptoms that provide a lot of expertise within the first few weeks in the onset of ketonemia. The same as the respiratory disorder, these symptoms will embody fatigue, brain fog, dizziness, vomiting, nausea, and abdominal pain.

The keto respiratory disorder - and also related to sugar cravings - usually leads people to give up the diet and start breaking down carbohydrates, but those who hold it out sometimes report that the symptoms disappear after many days or one or two weeks.

Before starting a weight loss program, you should consider:

Diets you've tried. What did you like or dislike about them? Were you ready to follow the diet? What worked or did not work? However, do you feel physical and showing emotions while on a diet?

Your preferences.

Do you choose to do a weight loss program yourself, or do you want to support a cluster? If you prefer group support, do you enjoy online support or face-to-face meetings?

Your budget.

Some weight loss programs require you to shop for supplements or meals, visit weight loss clinics, or attend support conferences. Does the price match your budget?

Other concerns.

Should one have a health condition such as polygenic disease, cardiomyopathy, or allergies? Do you have cultural or ethnic needs or preferences regarding food?

Make sure to select a draft that you swallow. Explore for these features:

Flexibility.

A multifaceted arrangement prohibits unbound food or food teams; however, it instead contains a range of foods from all major food teams. A healthy diet consists of fruits and vegetables, whole grains, low-fat dairy farm products, lean macromolecule sources, fruity, and seeds. A versatile setup occasionally allows for an affordable indulgence. It should contain foods that you will notice on your home market, where you can get pleasure from when recording it. However, the scheme should limit alcohol, sweet drinks, and sugary candies because the calories in them don't contain enough nutrients.

Balance.

Your arrangement should contain sufficient nutrients and calories. Absorb huge amounts of bound foods, such as grapefruit or meat, drastically cutting calories, or eliminating whole food teams, such as carbohydrates, will cause nutritional problems. Safe and healthy diets don't require excessive vitamins or supplements.

Likeability.

A diet should embrace foods you prefer that you will simply enjoy the shot forever - not the ones you tolerate over the course of the arrangement.

If you don't just like the food on the package, if the package is too restrictive or if it gets boring, you almost certainly don't keep up. Therefore semi-permanent weight loss is unlikely.

Efficacy.

Your arrangement should include physical activity. Exercise and fewer calories will help boost your weight loss. Exercise also offers varied health benefits and counteracts the loss of muscle mass that occurs with weight loss. And exercise is essential to think about maintaining weight loss. Before diving into a weight loss package, take the time to hear about the maximum amount you can get.

Simply because a diet is common or your friends do not mean it is right for you. First, ask these questions:

What is involved? Do you arrange the controls that you simply adapt to your situation? Should I go shopping for special meals or supplements? Will it provide online or personal support? Does it teach you the way to make positive, healthy changes in your life to help you maintain your weight loss?

What is behind the diet? Is there analysis and science to make a copy of the weight loss approach? If you visit a weight loss clinic, what experience, training, certifications, and skills do the doctors, dieticians, and alternative staff have? Can the staff coordinate with your regular doctor?

What are the risks? Can the weight loss program harm your health? Are the recommendations safe for you, especially if you have a health problem or are taking medication?

What are the results? What weight can you expect to lose? Does the program claim that you lose tons of weight quickly or that you target specific body parts? Will it take pictures that seem too smart to be true? Will it help you maintain your weight loss over time? Everyone wants enough calories to keep their body running properly. With any diet that you don't eat enough calories, the necessary nutrients can be harmful. Extremely low-fat diets can also be unhealthy for you. Everyone wants some fat in their diet; therefore, no one should be on a very fat-free diet. About 30% of the total calories should come from fat.

Some people start quickly because they assume that all problems in their lives are due to weight. Others have an environment of their lives that they cannot manage, such as Associate in Nursing Alcoholic Parents, so they focus on one thing they will manage: their exercise and what they eat.

Eating too little (anorexia) or only feeding tons to give (bulimia) are eating disorders. Some people found it tiring to regulate their diet. They will eat a lot of food, and they cannot stop (binge eating disorder).

Nutritional disorders are harmful to a person's health. Someone with an Associate in nursing upset requires medical treatment. If you can make changes, here are some proven tips:

Practice! Move every day. Walk to high school, sign up for a fitness category, and notice a sport you want / dance in your bedroom. It doesn't matter what you do - just move!   Drink fat-free, milk, or water instead of sugary drinks. Instead of three meals, 5 meals of fruits and veggies. Choose a range of supermolecule foods, such as lean meats and poultry, fish, beans, soy products, and nuts.

Eat whole grains (such as grain bread, brown rice, and oatmeal), which provide fiber to keep you feeling full. Eat breakfast. Studies show that individuals at the UN agency do breakfast higher in the classroom, eat less, and control weight.

Watch your portion sizes. Reduce output and choose smaller sizes at fast food outlets. Avoid supersizing, even if it seems a higher value. Taking diet pills and supplements is strictly prohibited because they are not authentic and can harm our body in various ways.

HOW TO IMPROVE INSULIN SENSITIVITY AND REDUCE INFLAMMATION?

Obesity-induced chronic inflammation can be an important part of the disease process of hypoglycemic drug resistance and, therefore, the metabolic syndrome. During this assessment, we tend to focus on the interconnection between mud, inflammation, and hypoglycemic agent resistance. Pro-inflammatory cytokines cause the resistance of the hypoglycemic agent in animal tissue, striated muscles, and liver by inhibiting the signal transduction of the hypoglycemic agent. The sources of cytokines in states resistant to hypoglycemic agents are the target insulin tissue itself, primarily fat and liver, but to a greater extent resistance to hypoglycemic agents (IR) may be a sophisticated condition involving 3 primary metabolic tissues sensitive to insulin, striated muscle, liver and white animal tissue (WAT) collapsed sensitive to the hypoglycemic agent and its downstream metabolic activity under traditional aldohexose concentrations. IR is closely related to mud, cardiovascular disease, hyperglycemia, polycystic ovarian syndrome, and metabolic syndrome (see glossary). Because the most important part of the metabolic syndrome, IR, is also closely related to the disease of non-alcoholic disease (NAFLD). The anti-lipolytic result of hypoglycemic agents is small in insulin-resistant conditions, which may promote vicious acylglycerol synthesis.

Another characteristic of resistance to hypoglycemic agents is an increasing discharge of free carboxylic acid. As we know, FFA can be chased by organs and accumulate as postural fat, such as viscus and internal organ lipids. And viscous lipids, as well as the deposition of acylglycerol, are involved in the pathological process and development of NAFLD. Many factors play a role in the pathology of obesity-related NAFLD, as well as complicated interactions between aldohexose and lipid metabolism, genetic predisposition, environmental conditions, and modulation of the viscous microbiota.

IR encompasses a good spectrum of conditions, such as faulty signal transduction of the receptor's hypoglycemic receptor and mitochondria, performing microvascular pathology and inflammation. Obesity, characterized as a condition of inferior chronic inflammation caused by overfeeding, may be a major reason for the sensitivity of small hypoglycemic agents, making blubber a significant risk problem for IR. Obesity additionally manifested as excess fat, arguably the primary reason for NAFLD, recognized as illness-causing physical injuries like steatosis and non-alcoholic steatohepatitis (NASH), and even carcinoma.

Blubber causes fat accumulation in adipocytes that activate c-Jun N-terminal enzyme (JNK) and nuclear factor-kappa B (NF-KB) signaling pathways and may later increase the assembly of pro-inflammatory cytokines such as neoplasm gangrene factor-alpha (TNF) - α) and interleukin-6 (IL-6). In most cases, animal tissue (AT) is a vital website for obesity-induced IR and can also have an effect on the liver and muscles through cathartic cytokines, as well as adipokines such as TNF-α. AT consists of many cell varieties. Among these, adipocytes and immune cells, such as macrophages and nerve fiber cells (DCs), have attracted significant attention as contributions linking inflammation to IR.

As a type of polygenic disease begins to develop, the body becomes less sensitive to hypoglycemic agents, and the resulting resistance to hypoglycemic agents also ends with inflammation. A regeneration can end, with additional inflammation causing more hypoglycemic resistance and vice versa. Glucose levels creep higher and higher and eventually lead to some kind of polygenic diseases.

Emotional stress can increase the level of inflammatory chemicals. However, it is not known whether stress alone will contribute to the occurrence of polygenic diseases. Inflammation (swelling), part of the body's natural healing system, helps fight injury and infection.

However, it doesn't just happen in response to injury and ill health.

An inflammatory response can even occur once the system comes into operation, while there is no injury or infection to fight. Because there is nothing to heal, the system cells that discreetly defend the US begin to destroy healthy arteries, organs, and joints.

Chronic inflammation has long-term adverse effects. So, the food you eat, the sleep you get and how much you exercise, they are all very important when it comes to the reduction of inflammation.

Inflammation can be a process that helps your body heal and protects itself from pain. Inflammation is dangerous when it turns into a chronic form

Chronic inflammation can last for weeks, months, or years - and should cause many health problems. That said, there are several things you will do to reduce inflammation and improve your overall health. Certain factors, especially the usual ones, will promote inflammation.

Consuming large amounts of sugar and high fructose syrup is particularly harmful. It will cause hypoglycemic resistance, diabetes, and distant scientists have also hypothesized that overwhelming heaps of refined carbohydrates, such as life personnel, could contribute to inflammation, insulin resistance, and obesity. What's more, ingested, pre-packaged foods that contain Tran's fats have been shown to stimulate inflammation and the epithelial tissue cells lining your blood vessels.

Vegetable oils used in various processed foods are another viable culprit. Regular consumption can lead to an imbalance between omega-6 fatty acids and polyunsaturated fatty acids, which some scientists believe may promote inflammation if you want to reduce inflammation, eat less inflammatory foods and supplemental medications. Base your diet on the whole of nutrient-rich foods that contain antioxidants - and avoid the processed products.

Antioxidants work by reducing the number of free radicals. These reactive molecules are made as a natural part of your metabolism but can cause inflammation if they are not under control. Your medication diet should provide a healthy balance of macromolecule, carbohydrates, and fat with every meal. Declares that you can also meet your body's needs for vitamins, minerals, fiber, and water.

One diet that is considered medication is that the Mediterranean diet, which has been shown that inflammatory markers such as C-reactive protein and IL-6A carbohydrate diet decreases, also reduces inflammation, significantly for people with rotten or metabolic syndrome.

What will the Associate degree medicinal diet do? Your system is activated as soon as your body recognizes something strange, such as an invasive microorganism, plant spores, or chemicals. This usually causes a method called inflammation. Intermittent periods of inflammation aimed at really threatening invaders protect your health.

However, usually, the inflammation, day in, and trip even after you are not vulnerable from being far away from the intruder. Then inflammation becomes your enemy. Several major diseases that plague us - including cancer, heart disease, diabetes, arthritis, depression, and Alzheimer's disease - have been linked to chronic inflammation.

One of the most powerful means of fighting inflammation does not come from the pharmacy; however, from the food. Choose medicinal foods, and you can reduce your risk of health problems. Systematically choose the wrong one, and you speed up the disease method.

Not surprisingly, identical. All foods with an inflammatory diet in the associate degree are usually considered dangerous to our health, as are sodas and refined carbohydrates, which are still meat and cured meats.

Unhealthy foods together contribute to weight gain, which in itself is a risk problem for inflammation. But in many studies, the link between food and inflammation remained, even as researchers took into account fat.

Anti-inflammatory foods

A medicinal diet should embody these foods:

- tomatoes
- olive oil
- leafy green vegetables, such as spinach, kale, and collards
- nuts such as almonds and walnuts
- oily fish such as salmon, mackerel, tuna and sardines
- fruits such as strawberries, blueberries, cherries, and oranges

On the other hand, drinks and foods that reduce inflammation, and thus chronic diseases. It should be noted that, above all, fruits and vegetables such as blueberries, apples, and folio greens are high in these things and are beneficial.

Research has also associated loco with reduced inflammatory markers and a lower risk of upset and polygenic disease. Coffee that contains polyphenols and various medicinal substances can also protect against inflammation.

Eat one dish a day.

Keep a pack or two leaf vegetables you need to provide your lunch bag and a cup of leafy vegetables or green tea to drink in all major useful dietary habits you can adopt. These leafy greens provide Associate in nursing medications with a double punch, due to antioxidants and bioactive compounds that reduce inflammation and prevent free radicals from causing new inflammation. Avoid getting hungry.

Skip the slot machine and low sweet drinks and prefer a high fiber snack with a little macromolecule like apple slices and spread, raw vegetables and hummus, or lots of almonds and cheese cubes instead.

The rationale is that feeding a balanced snack without extra sugars and refined carbohydrates are essential to keep glucose intermittently, traditional parameters, which successively help you avoid cravings, hunger, and irritability. Not only is this more fun for the people around you, but avoiding spikes and drops of glucose also prevents inflammation in the body, resulting in fatness, a type of polygenic disorder, cardiovascular disorders. Get to bed earlier, the TV and Netflix, and go to bed a bit earlier.

While looking a little indulgent, finding seven to eight hours of uninterrupted sleep is enough for adults, and we should aim for that as our norm. Usually, do not get enough sleep (six hours or less) causes inflammation - even in healthy individuals - the analysis suggests that it will increase the risk of metabolic problems, which will result in fatness, a kind of polygenic disorder and cardiovascular disease, further like madness and Alzheimer's. Stuff things up.

Look for ways to use a little garlic or herbs when you're cooking tonight. Perfumed and pungent herbs seem to have the potential to exacerbate inflammation, but analysis suggests they really do the alternative. There is even evidence to include garlic or herbs and spices such as turmeric, rosemary, cinnamon, cumin, ginger, and fenugreek, and it reduces inflammation that would eventually lead to cardiovascular disease, chronic brain disease, cancer, and metastasis problems.

Take a chance through alcohol

If you'd rather have a nighttime cocktail or glass of wine, consider abstaining for many days. This does not have to be long-lasting; however, excision alcohol briefly (while creating various medication diet and lifestyle changes) does help calm the body and reduce existing inflammation.

While analysis suggests that moderate alcohol consumption has some benefits, it is easy to cross the road from beneficial and anti-inflammatory to harmful and anti-inflammatory.

Anti-inflammatory diet

To reduce inflammation levels, aim for an overall healthy diet in an associate degree. If you are looking for associate degree consumption that closely follows the principles of eating medicinal drugs, consider the Mediterranean diet that is rich in fruits and vegetables, nuts and whole grains, fish, and other oils. The choices you make on the market will have an impression of the inflammation in your body. Scientists are still unraveling; however, between nutrition and inflammatory processes in the body; however, they understand many things.

Research shows that what you eat has an effect on the amount of CRP (CRP) - a marker of inflammation - in your blood. That as a result of certain foods would be processed sugars facilitate unharness inflammatory messengers who increase the danger of chronic inflammation.
Alternative foods such as fruits and vegetables facilitate your body's fight against aerophilic emphasize us, which can cause inflammation.
The good news: Medicinal foods are generally constant foods that will also keep you healthy in alternative ways. Therefore consumption with inflammation does not need to be refined in the eye or to be restrictive.

Simple rules of thumb for eating medicines:

Eat a lot of plants. Whole plant foods have the medicinal nutrients your body needs. So the consumption of a rainbow of fruits, vegetables, whole grains, and legumes is the best place to start.
Focus on antioxidants. They help stop, delay, or repair some types of cells and tissue injuries. Buy your Omega-3s. Polyunsaturated fatty acids play a role in controlling your body's inflammatory method and will ease the pain associated with inflammation. Note these healthy fats in fish such as salmon, tuna, mackerel, and even smaller amounts in walnuts, pecans, ground oil seeds, and soy.
Eat less beef. Beef can be anti-inflammatory. Are you a citizen lover? Strive for a sensible goal. Try to make your beef meal work with fish, crazy, or soy-based supermolecule many times a week.
Cut the processed things. Sweet cereals and drinks, cooked foods, and pastries are all anti-inflammatory offenders. They are high in unhealthy fats associated with inflammation. However, consumption of whole fruits, vegetables, grains, and beans can be fast if you prepare in advance for multiple meals.
Inflammation is part of your body's natural defenses - when a cut swells and turns red, it is inflammation at work that heals you. However, once it goes into overdrive, fueled by factors such as poor diet and smoking, it will cause a lot of health problems along with upset, diabetes, inflammatory conditions (including psoriatic arthritis), cancer, and even depression. Tame it in these

ways. Turmeric has a flash, thanks in large part to curcumin - a substance that gives the sunny spices its medicinal powers. In accordance with a recent review, curcumin reduces the assembly of a supermolecule that causes your body to overwork. Thus it should be worth asking your doctor regarding supplements. You won't be ready to get that much out of food (5 teaspoons of ground turmeric or two ounces recently has five hundred mg of curcumin). However, the spice's medicine potential remains a good reason to sprinkle it liberally over cooked vegetables or sip on those stylish golden lattes.

People every 7 days a minimum of five servings of peanuts, almonds, walnuts or cashews nosed, showed different results than those who did not eat them often, found a study at Yankee Journal of Clinical Nutrition. The medicinal effects of nuts are due to their dance band of fiber, antioxidants and polyunsaturated fatty acids and polyunsaturated fatty acids. Obesity - or even simply increasing associative waistline - is a major reason behind inflammation.

However, you can compensate for this by increasing your activity. A study printed in Drugs & Science in Sports & Exercise found that the smallest amount of inactive people had soil inflammation, although they didn't get slimmer. While getting about two 1/2 hours of moderate to vigorous activity a day, it included normal life activities such as gardening and household chores. Even performing a very small increase in activity tames the flames compared to the fact that the entire sofa is tied. It could just be a lack of sleep, causing inflammation. However, you behave when you are tired can also be what ignites the flames. During a study from Ohio State University, inflammation developed when couples with sleep disorders started to bicker. Once seen with a conflict, partners' inflammatory markers jumped half a dozen% for every hour of sleep, losing less than seven hours. Insufficient rest can make you very sensitive to ferret, which in turn causes inflammation—the good news: victimizing healthy conflict resolution provided protection for every partner.

Even if incidental is your nutrient, you may not need to make any tea at all, especially the inexperienced selection. The tea tray is packed with powerful antioxidants that ease inflammation of the quell. In fact, researchers at Texas University Health Sciences Center in Lubbock found that tea leaves inhibit aerophilic stress and, therefore, the potential inflammation that will arise from it.

If you drink one to three cups of low or alternative caffeinated drinks every day, consider swapping one for a cup of tea. Tea leaves are filled with polyphenol compounds, which can reduce nuclear damage to prevent additional inflammation. Studies board that is often drinking tea will promote back you millions of plug around probiotics, but do you support these sensible microbes already living in you? Defend those existing good microorganisms by eradicating extra sugars and Tran's fats and specializing in selecting mainly whole and minimally processed foods.

It's also extra-priced, overwhelmingly probiotic-rich foods - like yogurt, sauerkraut, kombucha, miso, or kimchi - every day. Strengthening the germ barrier of the gut is one of the cornerstones of reducing inflammation in the long term. Risk of Alzheimer's disease, cancer, and joint disease. Granted, it's not for everyone; however, the analysis continues to look for benefits once there is occasional abstinence (IF), especially thanks to the drug affecting absorption. There are many ways to approach abstinence, a simple thanks at the beginning; however, it is at a 12-hour speed. This suggests that if you finish dinner at seven in the evening, you will only consume water or black for up to seven hours straight. Research advisers who often do can reduce the risk of cardiovascular disease and improve endocrine susceptibility, brain health, and inflammatory internal organ disease. Notwithstanding, but healthy your diet, inferior inflammation is not abused as stress runs incessantly high.

And while stress is not an inordinate amount of daily drawbacks, learning how to manage and deal with it as soon as it arises is vital to prevent new inflammations—finding healthy ways to escape that stress - for example, through active yoga, meditation, or a short walk - provides physiologically rapid and anti-inflammatory effects physiologically.

WHAT IS NORMAL BODY FAT LEVEL:

No range can be a complete picture of your individual health. However, treating your mind and body are usually higher indicators of your overall health and wellness.

However, we tend to sleep at a time when doctors and alternative specialists had to use graphs, data, and alternative measurements to form a typical definition of health. That is why your doctor or health care provider can usually chart your body mass index or BMI during routine physics.

Additionally, while BMI and alternative measures like body fat content serve a purpose, it's vital to remember that moving your body and making targeted decisions about the foods you eat also contribute to your overall health.

With that in mind, consider BMI and body share only one with the notice of your weight, and given a BMI calculation is completely dependent on your height and weight, male or female makes no difference, but that range is calculated.

That said, there are differences between men and girls when it comes to body fat percentages.

 Body fat percentages for girls make up some totally different classes. Some charts can divide the odds by classes, such as athletes and acceptable ranges, while others divide the ranges by age. Being overweight can increase the chances of various health problems, including:

- type some polygenic disorders
- high force per unit area
- heart disease and strokes
- pregnancy problems, such as high glucose during pregnancy, high strength per unit area and an increased risk of cesarean section (C-section)

How do I know if I am overweight?

Gaining a lot of pounds all year round may not look like a huge deal. However, these pounds will add up over time. However, are you able to tell if your weight can increase your chances of developing health problems? Knowing 2 digits can help you see your risk: your body mass index (BMI) score from your authority's external link and your waist size in inches.

Body Mass Index

The BMI is a method of determining whether or not you are normal weight, overweight, or blubbery. It measures your weight in relation to your height and gives a score to put you in a very category:

1) Normal weight: BMI from 18.5 to 24.9
2) Overweight: BMI from 25 to 29.

3) Obesity: BMI of 30 or higher.

WHAT ARE THE RISKS AND BENEFITS OF THE KETO DIET?

If you explore the term "keto diet" online, you will see that there are several health claims regarding the ketogenic diet. However, before discussing the approach to this diet, it is essential to understand what science suggests regarding the effects it can carry on your health. You want to take into account the possible risks, as explained below:

Risk: you get fatigued and various symptoms from the keto grippe

One of the most common effects of the associated early ketogenic diet is that this term describes the usually unpleasant and fatigue-inducing symptoms that occur when the body goes from a diet high in saccharides to an occasional carbohydrate diet. Quite a keto grippe, the aldohexose donjon s in the body, begins to run, and also, the body begins to adjust to using ketones and supply as energy.

Symptoms of keto grippe include headache, fatigue, dizziness, trouble sleeping, palpitations, and cramps. These aspect effects usually diminish and eventually disappear over time. However, the consequences of any discomfort to illuminate, you just need to think about the transition to a ketogenic diet slowly instead of running to change your consumption habits.

By slowly reducing your saccharide intake, while gradually increasing your dietary fat intake over time, you can create a transition with less negative impact, and no doubt stop the keto grip. Risks include suffering from constipation.

"If you don't do it right - with most of your carbohydrates from fiber-rich vegetables - you won't get enough fiber, which could cause it," says Chris Mohr, Ph.D. ., a sports dietician, entirely based in the city, Kentucky.

Risk: You will most likely develop dangerous nutrient deficiencies

In addition, the elimination of food groups is going to be problematic. "Ketogenic diets are generally low in Ca, vitamin D, potassium, magnesium, and folacin, which over time, can cause biological deficiencies in the process if the diet is not carefully planned.

Risk: you risk damaging your heart by specializing in animal fats and proteins. Research shows that a diet made in animal fats and supermolecules can also have a negative effect on heart health. "This diet is not for people who are at risk of getting upset, or the administrative agency has already been diagnosed with this disease."

This means that if you have risk factors - such as high steroid levels or a solid story about the disease - you should be careful as soon as you start following them. Which is highly dependent on fats, significantly saturated fats can increase steroid levels, increasing your ability to develop cardiopathy in the longer term.

Risk: You most likely need dangerous symptoms if you have a genetic condition

For anyone with a genetic condition, it is essential to speak to your healthcare team about dietary changes, significantly as dramatic as those required by the ketogenic diet. Since carbohydrates in the blood are converted to aldose, removing carbohydrates from your diet can take place at an associate degree, quickly making a decision about aldohexose concentrations, betting on your current treatment regimen. Such a change would possibly as necessary changes in medication, and the hypoglycemic agent is to prevent dangerous facet effects like symptoms.

Risk: You will feel a weight cycle that negatively affects your metabolism

Aside from changes in physical health, one of the main problems with the ketogenic diet is also long-term compliance. "It is a very difficult diet to follow and maintain.

Compliance can also be challenging because it is therefore restrictive," explains Mohr. Follow display a strict diet, then quickly return to previous habits when dietary changes are too restrictive, which could lead to what is called as a result of the duty cycle of the art I fact. Weight gain or loss, time after time, has a very damaging effect on self and motivation. It will benefit you in a way that you will notice improvements in your athletic performance.

For athletes, analysis of the keto diet indicates possible improvements in athletic performance, significantly with regard to endurance activities. An article suggests that a ketogenic diet could potentially alter endurance athletes to trust wholly on their energy intake during the exercise, rather than supplementing with simple carbohydrates in the work and endurance competition, while recovery times.

Benefit: You're ready to freak out quickly, but in fact, not quite what you see from completely different diets. In addition, if you prefer to turn around, one of the benefits of the ketogenic diet is the ability to suppress craving. Associate research of this type of consumption suggests that it is intended to diminish desire, but the style in which it occurs should nevertheless be studied.

With weight loss connectedness, associate degree excess d attainable from the diet for many people, the benefits of the ketogenic diet will not really be completely different from the opposite diet. "This diet does not yield magical gains in terms of weight loss," says Spano. "The ketogenic diet can help you switch in a similar way to completely different diets, by limiting your choice of foods, so you eat fewer calories."

Mohr agrees, "Reducing the number of organic compounds can also be a huge reduction in calories," he says, adding that this result will lead to loss of water weight from the start, "which is why people like to respond immediately to their weight."

For a person who has diabetes, adopting a diet low in saccharide, such as the ketogenic diet, may provide some benefits for glucose management, for example, one study found that limiting saccharide nutrition could reduce the medication or eliminate the need for medication for people with some type of polygenic disorder.

Studies have shown that this diet will have positive effects on certain diseases as follows:

Heart disease: The ketogenic diet improves risk factors such as body fat, HDL levels, strength per unit area, and glucose.

Cancer: This diet is currently not suitable for treating many cancers and slowing the growth of neoplasm.

Alzheimer's disease: The diet will reduce the symptoms of Alzheimer's disease and prevent the progression of the disease. For example, patients who have epilepsy, the diet has played a major role and shown to have caused major seizure reduction in children with a brain disorder.

Parkinson's disease: A study found that diet helped relieve Parkinson's disease symptoms.

Polycystic Ovary Syndrome: The ketogenic diet can lower the endocrine levels of the shell, which can play a key role in polycystic ovarian syndrome.

Acne: Lowering endocrine levels and feeding less sugar or processed foods will reduce skin disease.

Ketogenic diets for polygenic disorders and prediabetes

Diabetes is characterization by changes in the metabolism hyperglycemia and impaired endocrine activity. The ketogenic diet will help you lose excess fat, which is closely linked to a type of polygenic disorder, prediabetes, and metabolic syndrome. In another study, the ketogenic cluster lost 11.4 kg, compared to 9 kg within the higher saccharide cluster. This is often a very important gain ever given the relationship between weight and type of a few polygenic conditions. In addition, 95.2% of the ketogenic cluster was together ready to stop or reduce anti-polygenic drugs, compared to 62% within the higher saccharide cluster.

Food to avoid

Basically, any food made in carbohydrates should be limited.
Here can be a list of foods to be cut or eliminated Grains or starch: Wheat products, rice, pasta, grains, etc.
 Fruit: All fruits except small parts of berries such as strawberries.
Beans or legumes: peas, excretory organs, etc. Low-fat products, including extremely processed and sometimes rich in carbohydrates.
Some spices or sauces: they usually contain sugar and harmful fats.
Alcohol: Due to the saccharide content, various alcoholic drinks are often harmful to you.
Diet foods without sugar: These foods tend to be extremely processed.

Food to eat

You should add these foods to your meals:
 Meat: especially red meat, bacon, steak, ham, sausage, chicken, and turkey.
Fatty fish: such as salmon, trout, tuna, and mackerel.
Eggs: look for organic.
Oils: especially extra virgin vegetable oil, copra oil, and avocado oil.
Low macromolecule vegetables: most inexperienced vegetables, tomatoes, onions, peppers, etc.
In seasonings, salt, pepper, and various healthy herbs and spices are used.

Recipes/meal plans

A ketogenic hotel plan for a week
To get you started, here's an example of a week-long hotel plan:
Monday
Breakfast: bacon, eggs, and tomatoes.

Lunch: salad with vegetable oil and feta cheese.

Dinner: Salmon fish with asparagus seared with very little butter.

Tuesday

Breakfast: egg, tomato, basil, and low-fat cheese omelet.

Lunch: almond milk, spread, chocolate, and a shake.

Dinner: store meatballs, cheese, and vegetables.

Wednesday

Breakfast: a shake

Lunch: Shrimp dish with vegetable oil and avocado.

Dinner: cheese chops, broccoli, and dish.

Thursday

Breakfast: omelette with avocado, condiment sauce, bell pepper, onions, and herbs.

Lunch: a few walnuts and celery sticks with dip and seasoning sauce.

Dinner: Chicken full of pesto and cheese, surrounded by vegetables.

Friday

Breakfast: Greek dairy product with spread, chocolate, and sugar substitute.

Lunch: beef sautés in copra oil with vegetables.

Dinner: bacon burger, eggs, and low-fat cheese.

Saturday

Breakfast: ham and low-fat cheese omelet with vegetables.

Lunch: slices of ham and cheese with barmy.

Dinner: fish, egg with spinach seared in copra oil.

Sunday

Breakfast: boiled eggs with bacon and mushrooms.

Lunch: chicken, cheese, and dip.

Dinner: sliced and eggs with a platter

Healthy ketogenic snacks

If you're hungry between meals, here are some healthy ketogenic snacks:

- Fatty meat or fish.
- Cheese.
- A handful of nuts or seeds.
- 1-2 hard-boiled eggs
- Dark chocolate 90%.

- Low supermolecule milkshake with almond milk, chocolate, and pasta.
- Whole dairy product mixed with pasta and chocolate.
- Strawberries.
- Celery with condiment sauce and dip.
- Small parts of leftover meals.

Tips for consumption with a ketogenic diet

It is not very difficult to follow a ketogenic diet. Most restaurants supply meat or fish dishes. Order this type of food and replace low-carb foods with extra vegetables.

Egg-based meals are a good option, such as a side dish or eggs and bacon. You can style any type of meat with cheese, dip, or seasoned sauce. For sweet, raise a cheese platter with berries.

Side effects and how to minimize them? This diet is usually beneficial for people in the physiological state; there are also some aspect effects associated with customization. This sometimes takes several days.

These are the most symptoms:

1. The decrease in energy,
2. The hunger will increase,
3. Sleeping problems,
4. Nausea,
5. Digestive discomfort
6. And a decrease in your physical performance.

To minimize this, you can go step by step. You can teach your body to burn a lot of fat before completely removing carbohydrates. A ketogenic diet can change your body's water and mineral balance, which will make adding salt to your meals or taking mineral supplements easier.

A ketogenic diet is not for everyone.

A ketogenic diet is recommended for overweight people who have diabetes / who want to improve their metabolism. Maybe less suitable for athletes or people who want huge amounts of muscle or weight.

And, as with any diet, it only works if you are consistent and respect it long term. That said, a few things have been tried well in the diet due to the benefits of the ketogenic diet.

Ketogenic diet and budget

The keto regime, while not breaking the bank, is it possible?

Because it is another problem of this regime that seems terribly fast, raw materials used in the menus are expensive: avocados, salmon, shrimp, seafood, duck, etc.

This increase in the average value of food in the future is to be qualified by the decrease in the amounts of the proteins, and in particular, the lipids make it achievable to achieve a lot of satisfaction quickly. There are cheaper products with which you can stay in a biological process ketonemia at a lower price.

Substitute product for the keto diet

Often sites and books that mention the ketogenic diet need a long state time change. And that we advocate that you just throw a fair bit of what you have in your closets.

Here are some ways to facilitate the daily ketogenic diet.

For a keto diet with a minimum of state change and solutions not to succumb to temptations, cravings for sweets, bread, chips, etc.

Low-carb and keto-compatible substitutes. There are several replacement products. The purists of the ketogenic diet usually discourage them: I believe that instead, they will be a precious help to turn life into keto, prevent squatting, and facilitate family meals.

You should look at the labels because a product sealed with a coffee glycemic index or Low Carb generally goes much higher than ten g of carbohydrates per hundred g. so do not trust and pay close attention to quantities!

It is possible to find:

1) low- carbohydrate food paste,

2) Dark chocolate bars and milk, with maltitol,

3) Ready-made mixes to make low-carb bread,

4) Ketogenic bread,

5) Low carbohydrate tortillas,

6) And even low-carb hazelnuts unfold.

7) Sweeteners

A family of organic compounds that are additionally offered in the form of polyalcohols is smart sugar substitutes as follows:

- Xylitol
- Erythritol used in baking
- Maltitol: used in low carb chocolate tablets
- and Sorbitol: sugar-free gum

The erythritol is usually the sweetener used in ketogenic pastries.

And to sweeten a candy instantly, there are blends of 50% Erythritol and 50% Stevia with the impact of neutralizing the false style of the 2 sweeteners taken individually. They are only partially absorbed by the internal organ, which may not affect glucose.

Is chocolate compatible with the ketogenic diet?

More than 80% of the chocolate is consumed in small quantities. If you swear by chocolate, it gets harder.

Ketogenic bread

You may notice recipes to make your own low-glycemic or Low Carb bread yourself.

Vegan ketogenic diet

Vegetarian and ketogenic diet browsed are largely for their medical benefits.

The ketogenic or keto diet can be a high-fat, low-carbohydrate diet that has become particularly known as recently. Despite the fact that it normally contains creatures such as meat, fish, and poultry, it is conceivable to regulate it to suit a diet for garden car enthusiasts.

WHAT IS THE VEGETARIAN KETO DIET?

The vegetarian keto diet is a diet regulating meant that consolidates elements of diet and keto, overwhelmingly fewer calories. Most vegans eat things like eggs and farm; however, maintain a strategic distance from meat and fish.

Meanwhile, the ketogenic diet could be a high-fat dietary routine that breaks carbohydrate absorption by up to 20-50 grams per day. This ultra-low carbohydrate intake causes ketonemia, a metabolic state in which your body begins to overwhelm fat as fuel instead of aldohexose.

With a standard ketogenic diet, about 70% of your full daily calories should come from fat, as well as sources like oils, meat, fish, and a full-fat farm. In any case, garden lovers' keto diet features meat and fish and relies rather on various healthy fats, such as oil, eggs, avocados, nuts, and seeds.

The keto diet for garden enthusiasts can be a high-fat, low-carb diet style that gets rid of meat and fish.

Medical benefits

While there are no studies that intersect the actual benefits of the keto diet for garden car enthusiasts, much analysis exists of the bipedal abstinence from food.

Progress in weight reduction

Both garden car enthusiasts and ketogenic diets are associated with weight reduction. An extensive survey of twelve studies was incontrovertible that those following a vegetarian diet lost a traditional 4.5 kg (2 kg) compared to non-vegetarian enthusiasts over eighteen weeks.
In addition, in an extremely 6-month study of seventy - four individuals with some sort of a polygenic disorder, garden truck lover diets shifted each fat and weight reduction extra adequately than standard low-calorie chuck less.
 In addition, a 6-month study in eighty - three people with heaviness discovered that a keto diet resulted in a notable decrease in weight and weight record (BMI), with a traditional weight reduction of thirty - one pound (14 kg). This gift feeding routine high li f e of solid fats may also keep you feeling full for extra wide to reduce craving and hunger.

 Protects against eternal ailments

Vegetarian lover diets have been linked to a reduced danger from some eternal circumstances. Indeed, they attach considerations to a lower risk of malignancy and improved degrees of a number of risk factors for coronary disease, as well as BMI, steroid alcohol, and wrist.
The keto diet has been to start d for its effects on disease compensatory measures.

In a 56-week study in sixty - six subjects, the keto diet prompted crucial drops in weight, complete steroid alcohol, beta-lipoprotein (awful) steroid alcohol, triglycerides, and aldohexose, which are all at risk for coronary disease.
Several studies suggest that this nutritional plan could protect the mind's prosperity and facilitate the treatment of Parkinson's and Alzheimer's infections.
Creature and test tube likewise take into account that the keto diet can reduce the chance of malignancies. In any case, additional analysis is needed.

Supports aldohexose management

Veggie lovers and keto abstain from food, any easier s aldohexose management. An audit of six studies linked garden car enthusiast diets to a motivational decrease in the level of HbA1c, a hallmark of long-term aldohexose management.

In addition, a 5-year study in a pair of 918 people confirmed that a garden truck enthusiast's dynamic diet reduced the risk of polygenic disorders by 53%.In the meantime, the keto diet can improve aldohexose guide your body, and increase its ability to affect hypoglycemic agents and endocrine working aldohexose management. In a four-month study out of twenty - one people, following a keto diet brought down 16% degrees of HbA1c. Amazingly, 81% of members had the choice to reduce or finish their medication for polygenic disorders before the end of the study.

Both garden truck lovers and keto diets will expand impress weight reduction, strengthening aldohexose management, and warranty against some constant illnesses. Keep in mind that no research explicitly checks the vegetarian keto diet.

Possible drawbacks

The vegetarian keto diet has a number of drawbacks to think about together.

May increase your risk of healthy deficiencies

Vegan diets desperately need to ensure that you meet your food needs. Studies show that these nutritional examples can generally be under minor supplements, as well as nutrient B12, iron, calcium, and macromolecule.

The keto diet for garden friends is significantly more and more preventative in light of the fact that it limits the number of supplements to thick organic process classes, for example, natural merchandise, vegetables, and whole grains - increasing your risk of lack of nutrition.

Carefully checking the absorption of supplements and nourishing an assortment of sound, complete nutrition will facilitate the guarantee that you are getting the nutrients and minerals your body needs.

Taking improvements can also facilitate - especially for supplements that are often unwell in an extraordinary diet for garden enthusiasts, for example, nutrient B12.

Can cause flu-like indications

Getting into ketonemia causes varied reactions, once in an extremely while

alluded to because of the keto flu.
Probably the most well-known aspect effects include:
1) Obstruction
2) Brain pain
3) Exhaustion
4) Resting problems
5) Muscle problems
6) Changes in mood
7) Nausea
8) Dizziness
It is noteworthy that these symptoms usually disappear within a few days. Obtaining much of the rest, remaining water-bearing, and active will usually facilitate your indications.

Not applicable to specific populations

Since the garden car enthusiast's keto diet is deeply preventative, it shouldn't be right for everyone. In're special, boys and girls World Health Organization pregnant, or breastfeeding has been forced to dodge it, because some indispensable supplements application will limit tie fulfillment and development.
It may also not be correct for competitors, those with a history of nutritional problems, or those with some type of polygenic disorder. If you only have basic conditions for your prosperity or taking prescriptions, talk to your health professional before starting this nutritional routine.

Canceled

The vegetarian keto diet can cause short reactions, wants important supplements, and is not allowed for young people and pregnant or breastfeeding girls.

Food to eat:

A hearty keto diet for green groceries enthusiasts should
include an accompanying assortment of non-boring vegetables, healthy fats,
and macromolecule sources, for example

- **Not boring vegetables:** spinach, broccoli, mushrooms, kale, cauliflower, zucchini, and bell pepper
- **Healthy fats:** oil, vegetable oil, avocados, MCT oil, and avocado oil
- **Nuts:** almonds, pecans, cashews, walnut on the bend, pistachios, and Brazil on the bend
- **Seeds:** chia, hemp, flax and pumpkin seeds
- **Nut butter:** almond, nut, walnut, and hazelnut butter
- **Whole dairy farms:** milk, yogurt, and cheddar cheese
- **Protein:** eggs, tofu, tempeh, spirulina, natto, and healthy yeast
- **Natural products** with little carbohydrates (with some restraint): berries, lemons, and limes
- **Herbs and spices:** basil, paprika, pepper, turmeric, salt, oregano, rosemary, and thyme

Short content

A keto diet for greengrocery lovers should include plenty of healthy fats, non-neutral vegetables, and plant macromolecules.

Nutrition to stay away from

On a keto diet with greengrocer and enthusiast, you should take your eyes off all meat and fish.

Carbohydrate-rich foods such as grains, vegetables, organic products, and soft vegetables are clearly allowed in modest amounts, as long as they fit into your daily carbohydrate indication.

You must remove the side effect of nutrition:

- **Meat:** hamburger, pork, sheep, goats, and veal
- **Poultry:** chicken, turkey, duck, and goose
- Fish and shellfish: salmon, fish, sardines, anchovies, and lobster
- Here are a few foods you should just limit:
- **Drilling vegetables:** potatoes, yams, beets, parsnips, carrots, and sweet potatoes
- **Sugar-enhanced refreshments:** pop, sweet tea, sports drinks, juice, and caffeinated drinks.

- **Cereals:** bread, rice, quinoa, oats, millet, rye, grain, buckwheat, and pasta.
- **Vegetables:** beans, peas, lentils, and chickpeas.
- **Natural products**: apples, bananas, oranges, berries, melons, apricots, plums, and peaches.
- **Toppings:** grill sauce, nectar mustard, ketchup, marinades, and an improved portion of mixed greens.
- **Well-kept food:** breakfast oats, muesli, chips, treats, waffles, and ready-made product
- **Sugars:** dark sugar, white sugar, nectar, syrup, and xerophilic plant nectar
- **Mixed drinks**: lager, wine, and improved mixed drinks

A yield lover keto diet knew all flesh that limiting high-carb nourishments tasteless vegetables, honey-sweet drinks, cereals, and natural products.

Test supper set up

This five-day take on getting the party started will help kick-start a vegetarian keto diet.

Monday
Breakfast: whole milk smoothie, spinach, nutty unfold, MCT oil and chocolate whey macromolecule powder
Lunch: zucchini noodles with tempeh meatballs and made avocado sauce
Supper: coconut curry made with vegetable oil, vegetable mix, and tofu.

Tuesday
Breakfast: Omelette made with oil, cheddar, tomatoes, garlic, and onions
Lunch: Cauliflower-topped pizza pie with cheddar cheese, mushrooms, tomato cubes, olive oil, and spinach
Supper: mixed vegetable serving with mixed vegetables, tofu, avocados, tomatoes, and peppers

Wednesday
Breakfast: curd scrambles with vegetable oil, mixing vegetables and cheddar cheese
Lunch: cauliflower macintosh and cheddar cheese with avocado oil, broccoli, and tempeh bacon
Supper: a dish with oil, spinach, asparagus, tomatoes and feta

Thursday

Breakfast: Greek yogurt with pecans and chia seeds

Lunch: taco lettuce wraps with pecans, mushrooms, avocados, tomatoes, cilantro, hard cream, and cheddar cheese

Supper: zucchini pizza pie pontoons with vegetable oil, marinara, cheddar, spinach and garlic

Friday

Breakfast: Keto breakfast cereal with hemp seed, flax seed, overpowering cream, cinnamon, and nutty unfold Lunch: Heated avocado barrels sprinkled with chives, coconut bacon, and bell pepper.

KETOGENIC HEALTH BENEFITS OF THE DIET

The ketogenic mold has been shown to have health and health benefits, including:

Decreased appetite and cravings: Different diets tend to let go of a feeling of constant hunger and misfortune, ultimately causing people to quit. The ketogenic diet is, of course, terribly fulfilling, and many people realize that they are not doing it to get the maximum amount of food or just to feel oversaturated. Individuals usually notice what quantity management they are developing and are now no longer tempted by sweet foods or foods as before.

Weight loss: reducing carbohydrates is one of the most effective ways to lose weight. Studies have shown that a diet containing coffee saccharides causes a few to three times more weight loss than a diet.

Improved blood glucose and hormone: A low-carbohydrate diet has been shown to reduce blood sugar and insulin levels significantly. Some individuals with the polygenic disorder may need to decrease their hormone dose by 50% within the first period. A study in pair 008 showed that in subjects with type 2 polygenic disorder, 95% had reduced or eliminated their polygenic disorder in six months.

Reduced visceral fat: Not all fats are created equal, and the fat in your abdomen called visceral fat is the most dangerous. Visceral fat is related to inflammation and hormone resistance. The ketogenic diet is effective in reducing this harmful fat.

Heart Benefits: a study conducted by a pair of 0 - 18 showed that patients with type 2 polygenic disorder some of their biomarkers valrisico annually improved from a ketogenic diet. In addition, vital changes in ignition and power per unit area were observed.

A keto diet refers to a ketogenic diet, which can be a high-fat, satisfying super-molecule, low-carb diet. The goal is to induce a greater range of calories from supermolecule and fat than from carbohydrates. It works by depleting your body from the supply of sugar, so the supermolecule and fat begin to separate for vitality, causing acetonemia (and weight loss).

A surprisingly common representation of a keto diet is the Atkins diet. Read on to familiarize yourself with the benefits of the keto diet.

1. Helps with weight reduction

It takes more work to convert fat into vitality than it does to convert carbohydrates into vitality. On these lines, a ketogenic diet will help speed up weight loss. Plus, since the diet routine is high in a macromolecule, it doesn't make you hungry like completely different weight management plans.
During a meta-analysis of thirteen different randomization controlled preliminaries, five results revealed a large reduction in weight of the ketogenic diet.

2. Reduces skin drainage

There are plenty of reasons for skin drainage, and one may be familiar with diet an aldohexose. Food worker eating routine with much handled and refined starch will change the gut microscopic organisms and increasingly cause sensational aldohexose changes, 2 of which can have an effect on the skin happily. Hence, by lowering carb admission, it is slightly, however, suddenly associating that a ketogenic diet would decrease some cases of skin drainage.

3. Can help reduce the danger of malignant growth

The ketogenic diet has recently undergone tremendous research on how it occurred or might treat linked malignancies.
A study showed that the ketogenic diet might be an inexpensive treatment equivalent to therapy and radiation in people with malignant growth.
This is often due to the fact that it can cause extra aerobic concerns in malignancy cells than in normal cells. Several hypotheses suggest that since the ketogenic diet lowers high aldohexose, it could reduce hypoglycemic agents, which may be associated with linked diseases.

4. Improves heart rate

When the ketogenic diet is followed with a healthy agent (which hinders avocados as solid fat instead of pig skins), there is some evidence that the diet regimen will improve heart rate by reducing cholesterin. One study found that levels of alpha lipoprotein ("large") cholesterin increased in principle in those following the keto diet. The LDL ("terrible") cholesterin went all the way down.

5. Can protect the functioning of the neural structure

More analysis is needed of the keto diet and also of the neural structure. Some studies argue that the keto diet offers neuroprotective benefits. These can ease or treat conditions such as Alzheimer's Parkinson's and even a resting problem. One concentrate even found that adolescents on a ketogenic diet had improved their sharpness and subjective action.

6. May reduce seizures

It is thought that the mix of fat, protein, and carbohydrates changes the way the body uses vitality, transmission over acetonemia. Acetonemia can be an increased degree of organic compound bodies in the blood.
Ketosis causes a decrease in seizures in people with a brain disorder. The jury remains informed, however powerful this maybe, but it is best for young people in all respects. UN agency has central seizures.

7. Improves happiness in girls with PCOS

Polycystic gland disease (PCOS) is an endocrine disorder that causes strengthened blister ovaries. A diet high in sugar negatively affects people with PCOS.
There are no varied clinical studies on the ketogenic diet and PCOS. A pilot study that included five girls over a 24-week period found that the ketogenic diet:
1) Comprehensive weight reduction
2) Helped the secretion balance
3) Improved gonadotropin (LH) / follicle-animating hormone (FSH) ratios
4) Improved hypoglycemic abstinence
5) More analysis is needed.
6) Hazards and complexities
The ketogenic diet can have medical benefits - along with a quick weight loss. In any case, it is important to require a note that the long term remaining on the ketogenic diet will have unfavorable results on your cheerful. These include an increased risk of:
Kidney stone development

Acidosis (significant amounts of corrosive in the blood)

Extreme weight loss or muscle degeneration (for long-term use)

Often quick responses from the feeding routine can include:

1) Constipation

2) Drowsiness

3) Low aldohexose

These facet effects are especially traditional at the beginning of the diet when your body changes. Your neural structure and your body's essential and favorite source of vitality come from aldohexose. On these lines, extraordinary sugar removal is not often a manageable technique for inner and ideal health.

Take

Any unusual change in your diet regimen can have potential results for your optimism. In this sense, you should systematically talk to your doctor or dietitian before starting a new diet.

In the event that you are keen on starting the keto diet, you need to be extra aware, therefore, seek the advice of your medical doctor in the event that you simply experience the polygenic condition, hypoglycemia, or coronary illness.

Since you don't want your body to remain in acetonemia for an extremely long time, you will point out completely different decisions for diet changes for the employee's timetable.

The ketogenic diet energizes the tip of refined and treated sugars. Be that as it may, not all sugars are created equal. Varied medical benefits come from the partner's diet regimen, including an assortment of supplements containing thick, wiry carbohydrates, organic products, vegetables, lean proteins, and solid fats.

There is a huge amount of messages, including the ketogenic diet. Some analysts swear this is the most effective diet for the vast majority to air, while others assume it's just an extra fad diet.

Somewhat, the 2 sides of the variables are correct. There is not one ideal nutritional regimen for everyone or for every condition, and it has little relevance to the variety of people who 'accept' it. The ketogenic diet is not a special case for this.

In any case, the ketogenic diet contains a lot of robust analytics to its benefits to support. Frankly, it is seen as superior to most diets in helping

people with:
1) Epilepsy
2) Type two polygenic disorder
3) Type one polygenic disease
4) Hypertension
5) Alzheimer's sick
6) Parkinson's is ill
7) Endless ignition
8) High glucose levels
9) Heftiness
10) Coronary disease
11) Polycystic ovarian syndrome
12) Fatty disease
13) Malicious growth
14) Headache
Regardless of whether or not you are at risk from any of these conditions, the ketogenic diet is often helpful for you, too. Some of the benefits that are excellent expertise from many of us:

- Better thinking
- Reduction of irritation
- An increase in vitality

The Calorie Mystery

Numerous analysts claim that ketonemia (consuming ketones for fuel) and sugar traps just take a small chore within the benefits of the ketogenic diet. Their rivalry is that, in general, people can eat fewer calories on the ketogenic diet, and this may be the first goal behind its benefits.

The facts show that people on the ketogenic diet can generally eat less, thanks to the satisfying intake of a low-fat, moderate-protein diet for the US. What's extra, it is the obvious starting that improves calorie usage prompts and improves cheerfulness and weight reduction; however, there is one thing that different scientists do not take into account.

The ketogenic diet calls for several important tools in the body and cells that don't exist in different weight management plans. These unique tools clarify the benefits of the ketogenic diet that fewer calories cannot absorb. The way the body responds to the ketogenic diet. A brief explanation of a way to adapt the body to the ketogenic diet. The purpose of the cell for reading

Starch is the body's favorite fuel supply. For the purpose, once its use is limited, the body reacts as if it were fast. This animates new vitality paths to enable vitality to the cells. One of these vitality pathways is called ketogenesis, and also, the result of ketogenesis is associated with elective fuel delivery called an acetone body.

These ketone bodies are often utilized by almost every cell in your body for fuel (apart from the liver and red blood platelets). However, sugar and organic compound mean acting upon the body from multiple points of the reading.

For example, intense sugar as a fuel makes more and more receptive element types. These responsive element types cause damage, aggravation, and cell death once they are collected. This may be the explanation that an excessive amount of sugar is thought to hinder an excessive amount of sugar and cause the development of plaque in the neural structure.

On the other hand, ketones provide more and more productive vitality and ensure safe somatic cell cells within the neural structure. This may largely be due to the fact that intense fuel ketones reduce the generation of responsive element types and improve mitochondrial capacity and creation.

The fixed cells that are trying to endure are also helped by the starch restriction. Although they do not have access to starch, a telephone procedure called autophagy is performed. This procedure allows for the up-management of various parts that improve cell size and strength, straighten the cell against damage, and evoke soothing shapes. The blend of autophagy and intense organic compounds is the foundation for serving people with malignant growth and mental health problems such as encephalopathy, headache, and Alzheimer's disease.

From the perspective of the body

Now zoom out and take a goose to; however, the ketogenic diet changes the body. Everything starts with an adaptation of the association in hypoglycemic agent levels.

By limiting sugars, we tend to take the best hypoglycemic trigger and out of the intake routine. These reductions in hypoglycemic agent levels build fat intensely and reduce irritation. The combination of those 3 changes tends towards the essential drivers of various incessant ailments - the opposition of

hypoglycemic agents, irritation, and fat accumulation.
Remove the mechanism from the keto diet from the start of the robot level, here is why the ketogenic diets will bring benefits stretching over the calorie restriction:

At the cellular level

Ketones consume extra effectively than sugar.
Starch entrapment causes autophagy and calming forms.
Consuming ketones as a fuel makes less receptive element types.
The use of ketones improves mitochondrial capacity and generation.

In the body

Insulin levels decrease because dietary sugar does not support secretion. Fat increases in weight precisely because the body has to use elective fuel sources.
Irritation is lessened with the argument that inflammatory fat levels drop, and less receptive element types are framed.
 The mix of the cell and also the substantial effects of the ketogenic diet provides the US with a reason why they could be useful in treating the conditions we have previously documented. In any case, this could just be natural chemistry. Is that the ketogenic diet logically irrefutable to help people with those conditions?
Treatment of encephalopathy - the origin of the ketogenic diet
 Our journey through the exploration of the ketogenic diet begins in 1924 with Dr. Russell Wilder. At the renowned Mayonnaise Clinic, Dr. Extra wonderful planned a starch diet to treat encephalopathy in children, and also, the exploration when it turned out that it had been extremely happy.
 The main top-notch study encephalopathy and the ketogenic diet was not paid until another time, in 1998. In this study, analysts noncommissioned a hundred young people, and almost all of them had multiple seizures per week despite taking in at least 2 seizure-reducing medication. The young people were fed a ketogenic diet every year. Lose your weight with the Keto diet
Ketone surface unit of the metabolic fuel created once your body shifts in fat-burning mode. Glucose and ketone surface unit of the sole energy sources at the service of the brain.
Consider ketones as a result of the auxiliary power supply of your body.

Before the advent of agriculture, when our ancestors were hunter-gatherers, they often fasted. The benefits of ketones return from your body and burn fat for fuel as well as the lowered aldohexose and hormone in your blood

The benefits of acetonemia include:

- Burn body fat
- Mental clarity and enlarged noesis
- Improved physical energy
- No sense of deprivation as a result of your expertise less hungry
- Stable glucose levels from very little to no intake of refined carbohydrates
- Skin improvements in people with acne
- Improved glyceride and cholesteric levels

Hormone regulation girl's agency of the United Nations continues with severe symptoms of PMS. Aside from the therapeutic benefits of ketones, many of us go crazy for keto because of the way they feel mentally and physically Acetonemia that eventually allows you to use fat for energy

The kids as ketogenic diet cluster significantly reduce the marker of hypoglycemic agent resistance called physiological condition assessment insulin resistance greater than those following a hypocaloric diet. An important marker for the sensitivity and disorder of the hypoglycemic agent, called high relative molecule adiponectin, multiplied significantly within the hypocaloric diet group.

2% of participants within the ketogenic diet cluster. Only sixty - two of the participants in the low glycemic index cluster. The ketogenic diet works for weight loss due to being usually based around a high-fat content, adequate macromolecule, and extremely low carbohydrate intake.

A high-fat, ketogenic diet is also macromolecule-sparing: your body continues to burn fat and does not treat proteins as an energy supply. Protein is also very important on keto. Ideally, you should consume 0.8 grams of macromolecule per pound of lean body mass. This can stop muscle loss.

For maximum success, start the keto diet using a plan that works for you. Determine how firmly you wish to push your body into a ketogenic state. A lot of sharp, you chop carbohydrates. The faster you are able to activate this method. Fasting is the quickest thanks to achieving a ketogenic state.

However, this could not be better for very every-day. For many people, a gradual transition to the keto diet is the easiest way to decrease on a ketogenic diet significantly supermolecule consumption forces the body to make changes to a unique supply of energy based on stored fat instead of sugars or carbohydrates. The body breaks down fats in the liver down to ketones, to which the most important is energy supply. The purpose of the keto diet is Triggering of a natural biological process to burn fat, achieve weight loss with a significantly lower intake of carbohydrates instead of cutting calories.

Here are the top keto supplements in addition to their planned features:
MCT oil.

This oil that contains medium-chain triglycerides will facilitate keto dieters add a lot of fat to their diet, and hold in symptoms. It is more digestible than old fats; however, it will have facet biological effects.

Exogenous ketones

These are ketones from outside of the door to provide as the opposition, of course, made endogenous ketones.

They will use an organic compound to increase blood and help in bringing home the bacon symptom rather .keto macromolecule powders—these macromolecule powders designed to have coffee carbohydrate content.

Keto electrolytes

Solution depletion is usual when the initial, start a keto diet because of water weight loss. Solution supplements prevent shortages of common electrolytes facilitating s as the metal element, potassium, and an atomic number of 12.

Digestive Enzymes

Due to the high - fat content of the keto diet, some people power expertise to facilitate biological process problems. The biological process catalyst supplements specific enzymes to break down fats. There are 7 main reasons why you shouldn't lose weight in keto despite your efforts.

You are not really in ketonemia.

Ketonemia is the state your body is in as soon as it burns fat as fuel instead of carbohydrates. Find out how you can inquire whether you have ketonemia and why secretion strips not tell as much as you think. You are ingesting an excessive amount in general.

Fat has a lot of calories, grams per gram, than macromolecule or carbohydrates. So you will be consuming a lot more calories than you used to.

Get information about calorie desires, additional because the ideal macronutrient varies keto. You have not been taken enough. Seriously limiting your calories slows down your metabolism.

You are ingesting an excessive amount of macromolecule. The keto diet can be a moderate protein diet, so aim for 20-25 p.c. of your calories coming back from macromolecule. You are intolerant or allergic to one thing that you take in. The main common food allergies within the US are to exploit for eggs, peanuts, tree nuts, wheat, soy, fish, and shellfish.

Food allergies and intolerances cause inflammation, which can lead to weight gain. You are leptin resistant. Leptin resistance is caused by irregular sleep, stress, overeating, and calorie restriction. Coincidentally, you can reset your leptin sensitivity with the tips below. Scroll down to see how.

The topics that follow the ketogenic diet:

Losing an average of 3.45 kg (7.6 pounds) compared to those within the UN Agency management cluster had no weight loss.

They lost an average of 2.6% body fat, while those within the management cluster did not lose body fat. On average, a few 3 kgs (6.2 pounds) of fat mass (the body part consisting exclusively of fat) did not lose fat mass compared to the UN agency management cluster. Maintain lean body mass to the same degree as that in the management cluster.

A high-fat, ketogenic diet is also macromolecule-sparing: your body continues to burn fat and does not treat proteins as an energy supply. Protein is also very important on keto; ideally, you should consume 0.8 grams of macromolecule per pound of lean body mass. This can stop muscle loss.

Since the decrease in aldohexose and an increase in the metabolism of fatty acetonemia brings a lot of benefits, the distinctive ability to induce weight loss is simply one that achieves acetone.

To achieve acetonemia, stop supplying your body with carbohydrates and sugar. This depletes your aldohexose, also called animal starch, and lowers your blood glucose and hypoglycemic agents. Hence weight loss on keto.

Your body starts to appear for an associate alternative supply of fuel (fat), releases it, and burns for energy. You want to balance the right macros, set realistic goals, and strive to get you closer to achieving your weight loss goals.

They had a very low intake of carbohydrates and macromolecules and, therefore, accidentally ran on ketones. Converting fat into energy is hardwired for our survival and natural part of human existence. Your body burns fat to use and produce ketones when the unit of aldohexose sources is low or depleted, such as during fast after prolonged exercise when you eat a ketogenic diet. Lipase (an accelerator which is responsible for the breakdown of fat) maintains the free triglycerides. These fatty acids get into your liver, and your liver and your liver turn them into ketones.

Much about this below in a way to look at the levels of organic compounds. Beta-hydroxybutyric acid (BHB) Not a technically organic compound, however, a molecule. The essential role in the ketogenic diet makes the scouting due to the vital acetone.

It enters the mitochondria and gets the adenosine triphosphate (adenosine triphosphate), the energy coin of your cells. Now that you just understand what ketone surface unit and the way ketonemia works, you almost certainly wish to understand why you should consider the consumption of a ketogenic diet, the diet that promotes ketonemia.

A ketogenic diet is an efficient weight-loss aid due to the dramatic decrease in carbohydrate intake that forces your body to burn fat instead of carbohydrates for energy. Results vary among humans due to many factors such as resistance to hypoglycemic agents and distinctive body composition, but keto has systematically resulted in a reduction in weight and body fat content in an extremely large selection of things but is not limited to the sorting of fat a few polygenic disorders and athletic performance.

To achieve the state of ketonemia, a metabolic state during your body for energy-burning rather than the intake of aldohexose macromolecules must be drastically reduced. The dietary recommendation that 45 to 65% of calories come from carbohydrates. One of the most reasons people don't smart down on the ketogenic diet is that they also have several different carbohydrates. In fact, only about five-hitters of your total calories need to come back from carbohydrates. It's traditional to own a touch issue surgery carbs times 1st to adapt to the ketogenic diet. However, to succeed in and maintain ketonemia, carbohydrates must be cut to vary the board. This can help you learn how different portions of carbohydrates you may own in a day while betting on your calorie needs.

Plus, consuming too many convenience types like hot dogs and food, once you're on the rum, will slow weight loss. These foods surface unit of nutrients - poor, meaning they are high in calories; However, few vitamins, minerals, and antioxidants.

Optimize your nutrient intake, while losing weight at the keto diet holdings with unprocessed whole foods. For example, full - fat farm product egg, fish, pastured meats, poultry, and healthy fats like avocado and vegetable oil surface unity all nice decisions.

Make sure you feature no starchy vegetables like greens, broccoli, peppers, and mushrooms to provide dishes with nutrients and fiber—Amount of calories you just consume or by spending a lot of calories through increased physical activity. If you turn to a keto diet and not pay attention to your calorie intake, you're likely to drop pounds. Because various keto-friendly foods, along with avocados, olive oil, full - fat farm, and whacky, unit area high in calories, are needed not to. Most people feel very happy when they consume ketogenic meals and snacks because of the filling effects of fat and macromolecules.

Scarce between meals is the produce of the calorie deficit needed to make slimes.

The ketogenic diet is a good weight loss aid. However, if you are having a difficult time losing weight, but you are doing everything right, it is a fair plan to rule out medical problems that will be prevented from weight loss success. These conditions will be dominated by your doctor through a series of tests. If you have any of the above conditions, don't despair. Proper management, along with medication, if needed, and modification and diet modification, will help you succeed and maintain healthy weight loss. It is traditional to require quick results after following a whole new diet; however, it is vital to lose weight will vary from person to person, remember. While the ketogenic diet promotes weight loss when properly followed, the rate at which you lose may not be fast, which is good. Small, consistent changes are the key to an off healthy way to drop weight and keep.

Not to mention using a whole new elbow fat routine where you lift a weight, you gain muscle as you lose. While these snacks are prudent, it's best to decide on lower-calorie choices if you're having quite one snack session a day. Instead of relying solely on size, measure your thighs and region of your arms weekly to track your progress. It is a good thing to eat healthy foods thanks to the prevention of hunger between meals and gluttony.

Nevertheless, some high - calorie ketogenic snacks such as the bend nut better, fat bombs, cheese, and jerky can also make your weight loss highland. Foods like non-starchy vegetables or protein will make you feel full of tomatoes lordotic in dip or a clouded egg with some healthy vegetables that make wise decisions for those following ketogenic diets.

Additionally, adding non-starchy vegetables to your diet adds fiber, keeping your system deuterium regular, which can be especially helpful for those switching to a keto diet for the first time.

Hypothyroidism, polycystic ovary syndrome (PCOS), Cushing's syndrome, depression, and hyperinsulinemia (high internal secretion levels) surface unit of medical problems that will lead to weight gain and build is difficult to change condition (5Trusted delivery, 6Trusted delivery, 7Trusted delivery, 8Trusted Source). While it will be tempting to pursue lofty weight loss goals, most consultants believe it is best to lose 1 to 3 pounds or about 0.5 to 1 pound per week (depending on weight) (9).), although slower, this can lead to weight loss, lean muscle mass, and reduce fat.

Transform your body and start a fat burning at a high level

As we should see, there is a unit of twelve basic laws if you want that area. Unit everything you want to remove that unwanted blubber from your middle metal. Most of them are powered by the unit; however, coaching comes into play. Your mass winning section is over for now; currently is the time to be too skinny.

These twelve laws of fat burning can get you there. Tap one is about simple math: you have to eat less calories than your body knows to drop body fat. Once a calorie insufficiency is formed, the body responds by creating it by removing it in body fat reserves to make the distinction. And presto, you grow shy.

All the different laws aside, this one is at the top of the list no matter which food approach you choose. Most boys UN agency surface unit quite active and exercise often burn with regard to eighteen calories per pound of body weight or a lot per day. It's basic, 200-pounder would consume daily three, 600 calories. To start with dropping body fat, cut your calories to between 14-16 per pound of body weight per day on exercise days, or 2,800-3,200 calories per day.

Dish dressings (low-fat/or lean dressing's area unit OK): remove the skin of chicken; replace a lot of protein for many of your whole eggs; prevent whole milk dairy farm products, and ditch marbled red meat like rib-eye for lean meat like flank. Staying perfect thanks to the management of these hormones is to control your macromolecule intake, as carbohydrates stimulate a hypoglycemic agent, an internal secretion that inhibits fat breakdown and stimulates fat storage. Some healthy fats in your diet Press fat store hormones, and you expect to soften a large amount of body fat away.

Eat fewer carbohydrates, and hypoglycemic agent levels tend to be moderate, resulting in fat loss. Of course, not all carbohydrate surface unit is equal. In short, fast-digesting carbohydrates tend to burst to form an oversized hypoglycemic agent, resulting in a lot of potential fat gain. If you usually eat a few cups of food paste at dinner, eat only one. Over time, you will see the consequences of hypoglycaemic management. Associate in nursing pulses does not lead to an abundance of a hypoglycemic agent increases, so they must conjure the vast majority of your carb consumption. The wisdom approach is to divide your macromolecule parts. If you tend to eat too big a beagle for breakfast, eat only 0.5 and keep the rest for tomorrow, or just eat a smaller beige.

As for carbohydrate selections, said beagle should be 100 percent whole grain and not white in every way throughout the day, in fact opting for whole-grain foods over refined foods, with the only exception being a physical exercise right away once it's fast - it carbohydrate digestion is supreme for boosting hypoglycemic agents and dietary fat, for example, is far more fattening than supermolecules or carbohydrates because it will likely be to build your body. Admittedly, carbohydrates are likely to make you fat; however, they additionally you're your coaching directly. Protein?

That's a good idea: it builds muscle.

Neither will fat; however, it is not useless moderate amounts of aid to promote dietary absorption and produce hormones. But if you're trying to get ripped, you should minimize your fat consumption. Protein, on the other hand, contributes not only to your key muscle by stimulating the metabolism, but will your metabolism really much straight increase.

 The body burns a lot of calories to process supermolecules, then it burns into carbohydrates or fat method, referred to as the energy effect of food. That's the main reason why diets that embrace heaps of supermolecule lead to greater fat loss than low-protein diets, even once every diet contains is a similar amount of calories.

We will not harp on this recommendation too: wear away than 1g supermolecule per pound of body weight per day. Your major supermolecule sources should be lean meats (chicken, steak, turkey breast, tuna), egg whites (the yolks contain fat therefore reject most of them as soon as you are making an attempt to lose fat) supermolecule powder (whey or casein) and lean farmers. Total daily caloric intake when losing body fat is hypoglycemic treatment crucial.

The total amount of hypoglycemic agent s freely through the body is not associated with just what percentage of carbohydrates you eat, however, how firm those carbs unit area digest.

Refined carbohydrates digest quickly and increase hypoglycemic agents well, so you should avoid them. However, if you do happen to eat, say a bowl of dry cereal, you will still take steps to confirm those carbohydrates to digest much slowly.

This can lead to the less hypoglycemic agent being free and, therefore, less control has far your ability to burn fat. One technique to slow down the digestion is to eat carbohydrates with the supermolecule and small amounts of fat.

Accompany that bowl of cereal, for example, with a white dish or farmers' cheese. Alternatively, you will eat a lot of vegetables, such as broccoli, cauliflower, inexperienced beans, and inexperienced salads, along with your meals. These foods really slow down the breakdown and digestion rate of all carbohydrates. Again, it's about hormones.

At midnight your hypoglycemic agent decreases sensitivity, which means that your body needs to unleash many hypoglycemic agent s than usual to put any carbohydrates you carry away the night to use within the body.

And right now, you recognize that higher hypoglycemic levels will decrease fat - burning and improving fat storage. In addition, the body naturally produces a thick liberating internal secretion at intervals of the first ninety minutes of sleep called somatotrophic hormone.

GH will not only burn fat but is necessary to increase the mass nevertheless creating and strengthening the system, and carbohydrates place a damper on GH unleashing, therefore, are ideal for traveling to bed under one in all 2 scenarios: Associate in nursing empty stomach, or even higher, only running supermolecule, no carbohydrates. This allows blood glucose, the refined name for digestible carbohydrates in the blood, to remain low, promoting the increase in nighttime GH production.

Not eat anything related to three hours before bedtime. A stronger possibility is for sleeping the ultimate four-hour meals to eat only supermolecule deal with one supermolecule meal immediately before the hour exclusively supermolecule as casein shake low - fat farmer cheese or pigeon breast fillet. However, you can eat a small portion of vegetables here. When we talk about fat loss and supplements, we sometimes tend to hear that fat burners are responsible for most of the energy you burn a lot.

The thing is theta number of side effects and perhaps disadvantages yet. Consider: it is a drug, it is there to treat health problems, but you are not sick, you are fat, and you only need to lose this fat around your belly.

Bodybuilders usually use it to accelerate fat loss. However, they collectively use many other things to penetrate there. That is a choice, but it is not going to be most effective if you are not set on an old-time expert stage.

Now there is a joint line of supplements that can act on glucose balance and internal secretion. Usually, work them through to glucose-lowering by at the gluconeogenesis work the method by which the liver of creating aldohexose from fats and proteins once no carbohydrate source unit area because of neither food or keep polysome within the body. Currently, we're talking, which is clearly the most important factor I would recommend to anyone WHO should start with a fat loss part.

One of the primary reflexes, once trying to lose fat, it is doing to cut down on the internal secretion output. This is often just the opposite of what we tend to do as soon as we need to make muscle. Here's what berberine can allow you to try. By lowering the total internal secretion levels, you can be in a very fat-burning state much more easily and for longer periods of

time.
It will collectively cause you a lot of internal secretion sensitive. That's the great factor with regard to it, as a result of you will be able to keep some carbohydrates in your diet and not only cannot it hinder your fat loss, it will make you fuller! As a result, you will be very sensitive, and carbohydrates are very simply driven to the muscle.

Generally, you may want less internal secretion to an identical amount of carbohydrates for your muscles to drive. Over time, this comparison results in a fuller l and less fat.
High hydrocarbons will result from long-term fasting, a calorie deficit that is too severe, an excessive amount of stress, etc. A sweat itself can be a variety of stress. Once you are fasting, you try to limit the energy offer out there; golf putting your body in a state of deficiency, which led can cause you to lose fat as the energy decreases the retention of energy, also known as fat.
 Because the energy is getting low, your body will not retain their need and part oxyacetylene. This method can be an n- endocrine hydrocarbon increase. Once this happens, within the end of the invariably elevated hydrocarbon, your body will push aldohexose into the blood by victimizing the method of gluconeogenesis. Is trying to lose fat, but it seems your own body is not allowing it, and it is fighting you?
Not really, because of a hydrocarbon is really very useful for losing fat. The hydrocarbon may include an endocrine substance that
Stuff breaks to energy to create and fight against unknown threats and external/internal stress. It also helps you lose fat because once it is deficient, it breaks down fats to provide energy. It increases internal secretion after your area unit understands; however, it can also break down muscle tissue if necessary.
The problem here is that individuals may tend to reduce their carbohydrate intake even a lot because they see no improvement, and therefore the method simply gets worse. You start to imagine an increase in water retention, feel puffy all the time, don't see any gains, and you're hungry like hell all the time.
Let's do some magic: per block, this method can not only give your glucose a lot of stables; however, you have simply found a weapon in the fight against the impact of stress aspect. So even if it's sensitive due to difficult secretion,

which is a formula for higher muscle growth.

A lot of carbohydrates in the muscle a lot of biological processes they will have a lot of muscle. Many female buyers are very happy with the impact it has on their cycle. It has produced convincing results in the development of irregular catamenia and ammonia in a group of girls with berberine for four months and a decrease in irregular catamenia from 15.3% pretreatment to 6.1% pos treatment. Of course, this study was conducted on ladies with polycystic sex complaints syndrome; however, even when not, we have seen some improvements in every cycle with its use. For girls who compete, mastering the cycle, and then adjusting the program, top of Form will be quite helpful.

Whether your space type is blown up to a level that has become a concern or you, have simply locked in the mirror and see you are a small amount much dad-bod than sex gods, the choice to shed a lot of unwanted pounds can be in the same shed measures dauntingly exciting.

Needless to say, getting more exercise can be a great way to travel. However, usually, forget that getting into a fashion modification can be that very often, your body is formed within the room.

Beginner or professionals, it is always wise yourself to inquire about some of the most important and effective rules for weight loss, so read on and see how to lose the kilos.

"Skipping breakfast won't help you change the state," says the NHS. Although there are several news reports to the contrary, a filling, early meal balance remains the most important necessary meal of the day. That's not to say you just can't wake up to your coaching with some morning fasting cardio. If you have a stable job, you are twice as doubtless to contract disorder as individuals with permanent jobs.

You are undoubtedly much doubt about cancer and fatness develop too. Your risk of polygenic disease will by no less than 112% increase, in line with a study. The only thing that results from your default position is to park it.

So when the opportunity arose to a bar table check to, I jumped (from the chair) on the possibility. Other edges are immediately apparent. I realize that I am extra focused on the task when I only know that every time I log in to the Facebook line or the Mail online, everyone will see what I am doing

Also, making the journey to stock in seconds is the hurdle to prevent you from having all you wish for. Many products can claim to be light, sugar-free, and low-calorie, but knowing the way to look on the other side and seeing what you really intense can help you avoid tons of hidden risks. One of the greatest tricks people fall for? Portion sizes. A bowl of cereal can say on the box that it's only a hundred calories per serving. H Court added the portions are too horrible totally different from yours. The nervous pig.

Fruits and vegetables, oats, whole wheat bread, rice, and food, on the side of legumes such as beans, peas, lentils, high in fiber. And why is it so important that we tend to you to ask to hear? Well, placing it alone is going to keep you feeling fuller for longer, while suggests fewer snacks and lower weight gain. Try to arrange your breakfast, dinner, and snacks for the week, so you can continue your calorie allowance, says the NHS. You might notice to create a weekly search list. This can allow you to control the spread of meals and ensure you are not caught and made to generate twelve parts of fish and chips. Inspect our meal school and batch cooking guides to get you started.

No one previously mentioned that this list was going to be fun. Again moderation is vital. There are different edges on the occasional nipple. Half of the added negatives of exaggeration could set anyone off. Amino also helps prevent muscle breakdown during cardio and stimulants. The system encouraging to many

Internal secretions to unleash, then much too energetic sources break and eventually some fat to burn. Sometimes you want this to happen at the end of a fat loss section if the energy restriction is high and you get stuck with the diet. For some reason, many people consider intense fat burners before even making any changes to their diet. That merchandise s embodies supplements such as ephedrine, synephrine, vasoconstrictor, and clenbuterol and Proventil.

Another family of fat loss supplements is a unit for those who act on the ductless gland. Kick-start fat loss intervals .skip steady-state cardio and alternating periods of full - scale intensity and low - intensity recovery. This type of cardio can ever burned calories rapidly hours after the exercise session is over. Increase your carbohydrate consumption when you are training and trim for carbohydrates when you are not. You do not compel to be at all nutrition pasta and bread from a cut to reduce undesirable weight. You just need only to be forced to your intake of macromolecules extra effectively to timing. Enter carb sport.

Carbohydrates sports can also be a more sensible approach than straight low-carb fast because it will allow you to keep a better course over time while providing the muscle animal starch needed to fuel an intense workout.

Proteins have a higher calorific result than carbohydrates or dietary fat, which means that you are in general less calories in the web store as a result of supermolecular prices, a lot of energy to digest, compared to 5-15 % carbohydrate and 0-5 % with fats. Super- molecule additionally has greater desire suppression properties, serving to calm your hunger pangs before they begin. Fasting as a result of too stressed berberine can work by blocking the method of glucose skyrocketing and can help you burn fat all day long.

So you thicken the hydrocarbon, but you don't get the rise in the glucose that blocks the fat burning method when you calculate, the amount you produce is much more than the basal, and berberine will not stop this. So, you have the possibility to muscle growth, while jointly serve your cells do some cleaning. Will even help some muscles to realize when you are sensible peri-workout nutrition received. Increase carbohydrates around the sweat, while you lot are internally vital.

Smart tips are with cheat days, not having tempting foods within the home, and not shopping for a family bucket, once a pair of wings would do molecule additionally has greater craving suppression properties, serving to calm your hunger pangs before they begin.

EFFECTS OF A KETOGENIC DIET ON THE HUMAN BODY

1. It helps prevent blubber

Obesity can be an essential condition that gives rise to various chronic illnesses such as heart disease, diabetes, high blood pressure, polygenic disease, and depression, which successively causes more problems for an individual. These conditions arise from a person's mood. The use of a ketogenic diet, however, can help an individual to penetrate to blubber and various related health problems to eliminate. Ketogenic can be a high-fat diet; therefore, using it can create an individual change status instead of gaining a lot. For example, using a ketogenic diet causes the body to burn fats instead of carbohydrates; therefore enables the reduction of fat cells. An individual will change state up to three times that of the person on an advised diet, other than the ketogenic diet.

2. It helps prevent polygenic disorders

Diabetes can be a disease in which a nurse has an imbalance between the internal secretion of the body and the level of aldohexose. A ketogenic diet will facilitate such health problems because it improves the sensitivity to internal secretion.
As we tend to mention, the ketogenic diet improves susceptibility to internal secretion, so in turn, it affects blood sugar. By keeping blood sugar levels traditional, a ketogenic diet helps you stop a polygenic condition.

3. It helps prevent heart problems

As we often say, it is a high-fat diet; therefore, it is an immediate result of the health and performance of the guts. Because the high-density lipoprotein improves and thereby facilitates the risk of hardening of the arteries and arteriosclerosis, these conditions cause the vital and major blood vessels of the body by the deposition of low-density lipoprotein.
The inflammation increases the pressure, and high blood pressure arises.

4. It helps against Parkinson's disease

Recent research has found that people on a ketogenic diet quickly eliminate Parkinson's disease. Some researchers claim that it simply helps reduce the intensity of Parkinson's disease symptoms.

5. It helps against presenile dementia disease

Alzheimer's disease is an Associate in Nursing acute disease that starts from a long time without symptoms, and once the advanced stage is reached, it damages the brains completely. The disease is only diagnosed in adult people because it shows no symptoms in the early progression.
Using a keto diet will ease symptoms and will help, to some extent, prevent this disease completely. The ketogenic diet converts fats into ketones in the liver. This produces energy that is supplied to the brain to form correctly and quickly.

6. It helps against encephalopathy

This diet was initially designed to treat encephalopathy in 1921. Before the antiepileptic drugs came in, the ketogenic diet was quickly used as a medicine. This diet is still used by many of us everywhere, the planet to treat encephalopathy and many diseases.

7. It helps against brain damage

The human brain can be a terribly delicate and important structure because it controls various or all bodily functions. Therefore it should be given the nutrients it desires. Facilitate the use of a ketogenic diet and to supply the brain with the nutrients it desires. Therefore, its use can facilitate concussion and brain injury.
Keto diet is the low-carbohydrate diet plan that aims to get more calories from proteins and fats and fewer calories from carbohydrates. The easily

digestible carbohydrates are removed from your diet, for example, sugar, pastries, soft drinks, etc.

This keto diet works in a way that it reduces carbohydrates and replaces them with fats. This process of carbohydrate reduction forces the body to extract energy from proteins and fats, and it begins to break them down for energy called ketosis.
 When ketosis starts, the body becomes incredibly fast to burn fats for energy. During this process, fats are also converted into ketones and stored in the liver, which supplies energy to the brain.
The keto diet has many benefits. It can lower sugar and insulin levels in the blood. But it should be remembered that this diet is only for weight loss and not for a healthy diet.

Why is the Keto Diet used?

This diet is actually used for weight loss, but apart from weight loss, this diet also has certain health benefits. It also helps manage epilepsy, heart disease, some brain diseases, and acne. More research is needed in these areas to understand better and apply. It is always recommended that you always consult your doctor first if you plan on starting a keto diet.

Keto for weight loss

A ketogenic diet is more useful and faster to lose weight than any other diet. You can lose weight from a keto diet for the first 3 to 6 months compared to the other diets. The reason for this may be that it takes more calories to convert fats into energy than it takes to convert carbohydrates into energy.
 Another reason may be that taking a high-fat and high-protein diet will keep you satiated and satiated for longer, which is why you don't have to eat for a long time. This is just an assumption that has not yet been proven.

Protection against cancer

Our body produces an insulin hormone that stores sugar in our body as energy. The keto diet allows our body to burn this energy stored as fuel quickly, so it is not suitable for long-term storage. This means that the body needs less insulin has and produces less insulin. This low level can help protect your body against certain cancers. It even allows your body to slow down the growth of cancer cells.

Protection against heart disease

Although it may seem strange to hear that diets with more fats produce good cholesterol, and diets with less fats produce bad cholesterol. Keto diets are not linked in this way. Keto diet does it in a way that the lower insulin levels produced by this diet help your body lower cholesterol, also by stopping your body from making more cholesterol. This ultimately means that you are less likely to have high blood pressure, heart failure, hardening of the arteries, and many other heart diseases. It is, although not yet confirmed, how long these effects last.

Helps stop acne

Keto diet also results in stopping acne. Carbohydrates are related to this acne skin condition, and in the keto diet, carbohydrates are limited, so it helps to reduce the acne problem. The lower insulin production from a keto diet can also help stop acne problems. Aside from the fact that keto helps reduce acne in the body, how exactly it helps has still not been confirmed.

Affects diabetes

Although the low-carb diets help your body to lower sugar levels much more effectively than any other diet. But there is a condition that cannot be ignored: the ketone diet, the body burns fat faster for energy, and when the fats are burned, it ensures that saved the connections of energy, which are called ketones. If you have type 1 diabetes, the higher level of ketones can make you sick. In this condition, it is better if you consult your doctor and adjust your diet to the condition.

To control epilepsy

Ketogenic diets have been believed to have helped seizures from epilepsy since 1920.

Nervous system disorders

Nervous system disorders are the ones that affect your spine and brain cells, as well as nerves, which connect both. The following are the disorders of the nervous system believed to be cured by a keto diet other than epilepsy:

- Alzheimer's disease
- Parkinson's disease
- Sleep disturbances

The reasons for this are still unknown, but scientists believe that the production of ketones through the breakdown of fats in your body for energy helps protect the brain cells from damage.

Treats polycystic ovarian syndrome

It is a condition in women when their ovaries larger are, and small, fluid-filled pockets will be formed around the eggs. This is due to a higher insulin level in the body. The ethical diet helps treat this condition in a way that helps lower insulin levels in the body. The amount of insulin you need and the amount of insulin you make, Keto Diet reduces both. So when insulin levels drop, this condition can also be treated.

Exercise
Exercises don't play an important role during a keto diet. It can only help with exercise, but it does not fit well with the full exercises, as they are beneficial during other diet plans.

Side effects of Keto

With the many benefits, the keto diet can also have its side effects. The most common side effects are constipation, digestive disorders, low or mild blood pressure. These are not serious.
Kidney stones and a lot of acid in your body are the serious side effects of keto, which result from low-carb diets. Other than this, the side effect also includes keto flu. It includes weakness, headache, irritation, fatigue, and bad breath.

Instructions for diet

It is always recommended to start and stop a diet plan according to your doctor's guidelines. Because when the body burns stored fat for energy purposes, then it becomes a burden on your kidneys. It is always challenging and difficult to start a diet and then switch to normal, especially if you have diseases such as diabetes, heart disease, or blood pressure problems.
This is the introduction of the keto diet that what it is, and what are the benefits and side effects. We will now briefly discuss the types of keto and some dietary suggestions you should take and what you should not eat on a keto diet.

Kinds of a ketogenic diet

There are mainly four different types of the keto diet, which are as follows.

Standard ketogenic diet

Abbreviated as SKD, this is a very low-carbohydrate diet with modest protein content and high fats. It usually contains 5% carbohydrates, 20% proteins, and 75% fats.

Cyclic ketogenic diet

Abbreviated as CKD, this type of diet plan means that the carbohydrates are reused after certain periods. For example, 2 carbohydrate-rich days after the 5 ketogenic days

Targeted ketogenic diet

Abbreviated as TKD, this type of diet allows the person to add carbohydrates after training exercises.

Protein-rich ketogenic diet

This kind of keto diet is similar to the standard ketogenic diet but differs in that it contains higher protein content. In this diet, the ratio is 5% carbohydrates, 35% proteins, and 60% fats.

Only two of these species have to date been studied in-depth and detail. These are standard ketogenic diet and high protein ketogenic diet. The other two are just advanced methods and are used only by athletes and bodybuilders.

WHICH FOODS TO AVOID IN KETOGENIC DIETS

The foods that contain high carbohydrates should be avoided in the ketogenic diet. Below is the list of foods that should be limited during the keto diet.

- Sugary food
- Grains or starch
- Fruit
- Beans or legumes
- Root vegetables and tubers
- Low-fat or diet products
- Spices or sauces
- Unhealthy fats
- Alcohol
- Sugar free diet food

Which foods to eat in the ketogenic diet

During the ketogenic diet, those meals should be eaten, including the following foods:

- ✓ Meat
- ✓ Fat fish
- ✓ Egg
- ✓ Butter and cream
- ✓ Unprocessed cheese
- ✓ Nuts and seeds
- ✓ Healthy oils
- ✓ Avocados
- ✓ Low-carb vegetables
- ✓ Spices

What are the healthy snacks?

Below is the list of some approved snacks that you can take if you are hungry during a ketogenic diet:
Fatty meat or fish

Cheese
A handful of nuts or seeds
Cheese with olives
1–2 Hard-boiled eggs
90% dark chocolate
Low-carbohydrate milkshake
Full-fat yogurt
Strawberries with whipped cream
Celery with Salsa and Guacamole
Smaller portions of leftover meals

21 Day Keto Diet Weight Loss Meal Plan

Does the meal plan have some pointers on how to use this ketogenic diet?
 Every day, the calorie intake is designed for 1500 to 1700 calories, which is designed for weight loss. The ingredients and quantity for this plan are designed for one person. If you want to add more people, multiply the quantities. You can replace any recipe and ingredient from your diet, and you just need to calculate the number of calories. It is recommended to follow this diet plan strictly.

WEEK 1

	Breakfast	Lunch	Supper	Total number of instructions
Sunday	chorizo Ontbijtbak	Sesame Pork Lettuce wraps	Avocado Lime Salmon	Calories: 1,520 Fat: 109g Protein: 110g Net carbohydrates: 16 g
Monday	Leftover r Chorizo Breakfast Bak with 3- slices thick-sliced bacon	Spiced pumpkin soup	Leftover avocado-lime salmon	Calories: 1,570 Fat: 124 g Protein: 92g Net carbohydrates: 16 g
Tuesday	Fried eggs in avocado	Easy beef curry	Rosemary roasted chicken and vegetables	Calories: 1,700 Fat: 128.5 g Protein: 103 g Net carbohydrates: 22 g
Wed.	Lemon Poppy Ricotta Pancakes with 3 slices of thick-cut bacon	Leftover spiced pumpkin soup with ½ medium	Leftover rosemary roasted chicken and vegetables	Calories: 1,665 Fat: 130 g Protein: 95.5 g Net carbohydrates: 23.5 g

		avocado		
Thursday	Leftover Lemon Poppy Ricotta Pancakes with 3 slices of thick-cut bacon	Leftover spiced pumpkin soup	Cheesy Sausage Mushroom Skillet with- 1 Slice Thick-Cut Bacon	Calories: 1,650 Fat: 126g Protein: 100.5 g Net carbohydrates: 22.5 g
Friday	Sweet blueberry coconut porridge with 1 slice of thickly sliced bacon	Leftover Easy Beef Curry	Leftover Cheesy Sausage Mushroom Skillet	Calories: 1,670 Fat: 112g Protein: 100g Net carbohydrates: 33.5 g
Saturday	Leftover Sweet Blueberry Coconut Porridge	Leftover Easy Beef Curry	Lamb chops with rosemary and garlic	Calories: 1,625 Fat: 108g Protein: 110.5 g Net carbohydrates: 27 g

Chorizo Breakfast box

Ingredients

- 1 tablespoon of olive oil
- ½ cup chopped red bell pepper
- ½ cup chopped yellow onion
- 4 ounces chorizo sausage
- Two large eggs
- Salt and pepper
- 2 slices of thick-cut bacon (cooked)

Instructions

Firstly, preheat the oven to 350-degrees. Now take two baking dishes and lightly grease them. Then heat the oil in a skillet over medium heat. Then add the chopped peppers and onions. Cook for 4 to 5 minutes until browned. Divide this cooked vegetable mixture between the two baking dishes. Chop the chorizo sausages and divide them too. Break an egg into each baking dish and season with salt and pepper. Bake for 10 to 12 minutes. Then crumble the bacon on the top and serve.

Fried eggs in avocado

Ingredients

- 1 piece of a medium avocado
- 2 tbsp. lime juice
- 2 large eggs
- Salt and pepper
- 2 tablespoons cheddar cheese (shredded)

Instructions

Preheat the oven to 450 ° F. Take the avocado and cut it in half. After cutting, scoop out the avocado. Place these avocado halves upright in a baking dish and brush thoroughly with lime juice. Now break an egg into each half and season with salt and pepper. Bake them for 10 minutes and add cheese. Bake the eggs for 2 to 3 minutes until the cheese has melted. Serve them hot.

Lemon Poppy Ricotta Pancakes

Ingredients

- 1 large lemon

- 6 ounces whole milk ricotta
- 3 large eggs
- 10 to 12 drops of liquid stevia
- ¼ cup of almond flour
- 1 cup of egg white protein powder
- 1 tablespoon of poppy seeds
- ¾ teaspoons of baking powder
- ¼ cup powdered erythritol
- 1 tablespoon of whipped cream

Instructions

Place the eggs, ricotta, and liquid stevia in a blender with half of the lemon juice and lemon zest. Mix them well and put them in a bowl. Now beat the almond flour, egg white powder, poppy seeds, baking powder, and a pinch of salt and put them in the bowl.

Now take a large nonstick pan and heat it over medium heat. Take about ¼ cup of batter and add pancakes. Cook these pancakes until air bubbles form on the surface, then turn them over. Now also cook the other side until brown and make the others like that. Beat the cream, erythritol powder, and the remaining lemon juice and lemon zest. Serve the pancakes warm and sprinkle them with the lemon glaze.

Sweet blueberry coconut porridge

Ingredients

- 1 cup of unsweetened almond milk
- ¼ cup of canned coconut milk
- ¼ cup of coconut flour
- ¼ cup of grounded linseed
- 1 teaspoon of ground cinnamon
- ¼ teaspoon of ground nutmeg
- Squeeze salt
- 60 grams of blueberries
- ¼ cup of shaved coconut

Instructions

Heat both the almond and coconut milk in a pan over low heat. Beat the coconut flour, linseed, cinnamon, nutmeg, and salt in the milk. Now increase the heat and cook until the mixture starts to bubble. Add the sweetener and vanilla extract and cook until the mixture thickens to the desired level.

Take two bowls before serving and transfer the prepared porridge into it. Top with blueberries and shaved coconut.

Sesame Pork Lettuce Wraps

Ingredients

- 1 tablespoon of olive oil
- ¼ cup of chopped yellow onion
- ¼ cup chopped green pepper
- 2 tablespoons of chopped celery
- 6 grams of ground pork
- ¼ teaspoon of onion powder
- ¼ teaspoon of garlic powder
- 2 tablespoons of soy sauce
- 1 teaspoon of sesame oil
- 4 leaves of butter lettuce
- 1 tablespoon of toasted sesame seeds

Instructions

Take the oil in a frying pan and heat it over medium heat. Then add the onions, peppers, and celery when the oil is heated and fry for 5 minutes. Now add the pork and cook until light brown. Now add the onion powder and garlic powder. Stir in the soy sauce and sesame oil. Season with salt and pepper to taste, then remove from the heat. Take the separated lettuce leaves on a plate and spread the pork mixture evenly with a spoon. Sprinkle with sesame seeds and serve.

Spiced pumpkin soup

Ingredients

- 2 tablespoons of unsalted butter
- 1 small chopped yellow onion
- 2 cloves of crushed garlic
- 1 teaspoon of ground ginger
- ½ teaspoon of cinnamon powder
- ¼ teaspoon powdered nutmeg

- Salt and pepper to taste
- ½ cup of pumpkin puree
- 1 cup of chicken stock
- 3 slices of thick-cut bacon
- ¼ cup of whipped cream

Instructions

Take a large saucepan, melt the but to over medium heat. Then add the onions, garlic, and ginger and cook for 3 to 4 minutes until the onions are translucent. Add the spices and cook for 1 minute until fragrant. Season with salt and pepper. Now is the time for the pumpkin puree and chicken broth add to. Bring them to a boil.

Now reduce the heat and simmer for 20 minutes, then remove from the heat. Mix the soup well with a hand blender and then put it back on the stove and simmer for 20 minutes—Cook the bacon crispy.

To remove the excess oil, place these bacon strips on a paper towel. Add the bacon fat and the cream to the soup. Now crumble the bacon over it and serve.

Easy beef curry

Ingredients

- 1 medium chopped yellow onion
- One tablespoon of crushed garlic
- One tablespoon of grated ginger
- One and ¼ cups of canned coconut milk
- 1 pound chopped beef head
- 2 tablespoons of curry powder
- 1 teaspoon of salt
- ½ c freshly cut cilantro

Instructions

Add the onion, garlic, and ginger in a blender and mix well to form a paste. Take a pan and bring the past one in it, then cook for 3 minutes over medium heat. Now add the coconut milk and let it simmer gently for 10 minutes. Then add the minced beef together with the curry powder and the salt. Stir well, cover, and simmer for 20 minutes. Remove the lid and simmer for another 20 minutes until the beef is cooked through. Season to taste and garnish with freshly chopped cilantro.

Avocado Lime Salmon

Ingredients

- 100 grams of chopped cauliflower
- 1 large avocado
- One tablespoon of fresh lime juice
- 2 tablespoons of chopped red onion
- 2 tablespoons of olive oil
- Two boneless salmon fillets
- Salt and pepper

Instructions

Take a blender and mix the cauliflower into rice-like grains. Now take a frying pan and grease it with cooking spray. Heat the skillet over medium heat. Now add the rice-like cauliflower, cover, and sauté for 8 minutes. Set it aside. Now well-assembled over the avocado, lime juice, and red onion in a food processor. Take a large skillet and heat the olive oil over medium heat. Take the salmon and season with salt and pepper. Then add the seasoned salmon skin side down.

Cook for 4 to 5 minutes per side until browning, then turn over and cook for another 4 to 5 minutes. Now serve the salmon on a bed of cauliflower rice and top with the avocado cream.

Rosemary roasted chicken and vegetables

Ingredients

- 4 pieces of boneless chicken thighs
- Salt and pepper
- 1 small sliced zucchini
- Two small peeled and sliced carrots
- One small peeled and sliced parsnip
- 2 cloves of sliced garlic
- 3 tablespoons of olive oil

- One tablespoon of balsamic vinegar
- Two teaspoons freshly cut rosemary

Instructions

Preheat the oven to 350 ° F. Take a small rimmed baking sheet and lightly grease it with cooking spray. Peel the chicken thighs with salt and pepper and place on the baking tray. Place the vegetables around the chicken and sprinkle with sliced garlic. Now beat the remaining ingredients together and sprinkle over the chicken and vegetables. Bake them for 30 minutes and then roast for 3 to 5 minutes until the skin is crispy.

Cheesy Sausage and Mushroom Skillet

Ingredients

- 1 tablespoon of coconut oil
- 6 ounces of Italian sausage, crumbled
- 4 ounces sliced mushrooms
- 1 small yellow onion, finely chopped
- ½ teaspoon of dried oregano
- ¼ teaspoon of dried thyme
- Salt and pepper
- ¼ cup of Marinara sauce
- ¼ cup of water
- ½ cup of grated mozzarella

Instructions

Preheat your oven to 350 ° F. Take a large cast-iron skillet and heat the oil over medium heat until it starts to smoke. Now add the sausages to the heated oil and cook them until brown and almost cooked through. Now remove the sausages and let them cool for a few minutes. Then add the mushrooms and onions to the pan and cook for 3 to 4 minutes until browned. Now slice the sausages and put them back in the pan. Sprinkle the oregano, thyme, salt, and pepper. Add in the sauce and water, and stir well. Now transfer the skillet to the oven and cook for another 10 minutes. Add the mozzarella and cook for another 5 minutes until the cheese has melted.

WEEK 2

	Breakfast	Lunch	Supper	Total number of instructions
Sunday	Fat busting vanilla protein smoothie	Easy Cheese Burger Salad	Chicken Zoodle Alfredo	Calories: 1,530 Fat: 113.5 g Protein: 107 g Net carbohydrates: 18.5 g
Monday	Savory ham and cheese waffles with two slices of thickly sliced bacon	Pan-Fried Pepperoni Pizzas	Cabbage and sausage skillet	Calories: 1,670 Fat: 129g Protein: 103g Net carbohydrates: 20.5 g
Tuesday	Mozzarella Veggie-Loaded Quiche with- 1 slice thick-sliced bacon	Leftover easy cheeseburger salad	Gyro salad with Avo-Tzatziki	Calories: 1,580 Fat: 104.5 g Protein: 117 g net carbohydrates: 33 g
Wed.	Pepper Jack Sausage Egg muffins with 3 slices of thick-cut bacon	Leftover Pan-Fried Pepperoni Pizza	Leftover cabbage and sausage skillet	Calories: 1,650 Fat: 127.5 g Protein: 101 g Net carbohydrates: 29 g

Thursday	Leftover Savory Ham and Cheese Waffles with- 1 Slice Thick-Cut Bacon	Leftover cabbage and sausage skillet	Leftover Chicken Zoodle Alfredo	Calories: 1,620 Fat: 119g Protein: 119g Net carbohydrates: 18.5 g
Friday	Leftover Pepper Jack Sausage Egg muffins with 1 slice of thick-cut bacon	Leftover Pan-Fried Pepperoni Pizza	Leftover gyro salad with Avo-Tzatziki	Calories: 1,595 Fat: 116g Protein: 110g Net carbohydrates: 15.5 g
Saturday	Leftover Pepper Jack Sausage Egg muffins with ½ medium avocado	Leftover cabbage and sausage skillet with one slice of thickly sliced bacon	Leftover gyro salad with Avo-Tzatziki	Calories: 1605 Fat: 118.5g Protein: 102g Net carbohydrates: 22.5 g

Fat busting vanilla protein smoothie
Ingredients

- One scoop of vanilla protein powder

* ½ cup of whipped cream
* ¼ cup of vanilla almond milk
* Four ice cubes
* 1 tablespoon of coconut oil
* 1 tablespoon of powdered erythritol
* ½ teaspoon vanilla extract
* ¼ cup of whipped cream

Instructions

Combine all ingredients in a blender except the cream and mix well. Blend them for about 30 to 60 seconds until smooth. Pour the blended shake into a glass and cover with whipped cream.

Savory Ham and Cheese Waffles

Ingredients

* Four large eggs
* Two balls of protein powder
* 1 teaspoon of baking powder
* 1/3 cup of melted butter
* ½ teaspoon of salt
* 1 ounce of chopped ham
* ¼ cup of grated cheddar cheese

Instructions

Take two eggs and separate the other two and set them aside. Now beat the egg yolks of two eggs with the egg white powder, baking powder, butter, and salt in a mixing bowl. Now fold the finely chopped ham and grated cheddar cheese into the beaten egg yolks. Then beat the egg white in a separate bowl and add a pinch of salt. Mix the egg yolks with proteins by gentle folding of the mixture and then dividing into two batches. Now grease a preheated waffle iron with cooking spray and spoon in ¼ cup of batter and close it. Cook until the wafer is golden brown, then remove for about 2 to 3 minutes.

Make the leftover waffles in the same way and heat the oil in a frying pan while frying the eggs with salt and pepper. Now serve the waffles warm, topped with a fried egg.

Pepper Jack Sausage Egg Muffins

Ingredients

- 10 grams of ground breakfast sausage
- ½ cup chopped yellow onion
- ¼ teaspoon of garlic powder
- Salt and pepper
- 3 large beaten eggs
- 2 tablespoons of whipped cream
- ½ cup of grated pepper cheese

Instructions

At first, make sure to preheat the oven to 350 degrees. Then lightly grease three baking trays with cooking spray. Mix the ground sausage, chopped onion, garlic powder, salt, pepper, and in a mixing bowl. Spread the sausage mixture evenly on the baking trays. Make a hole in the center by spreading the mixture over the sides. Now beat the eggs and whipped cream together with salt and pepper. Now divide the egg mixture into the sausage cups and cover with grated cheese. Bake for 25 to 30 minutes until the eggs set, and the cheese is browned.

Easy cheeseburger salad

Ingredients

- 7 grams of minced meat
- Salt and pepper
- Three tablespoons of mayonnaise
- One tablespoon of chopped pickles
- 1 teaspoon of mustard
- ½ teaspoon of ketchup
- Pinch of smoked paprika
- 3 ounces chopped romaine lettuce
- 1/3 cup chopped tomatoes
- ¼ cup of grated cheddar cheese

Instructions

First, heat the minced meat and fry it on high heat until brown. When the meat is browned, season with salt and pepper to taste. Now drain the fat separated from beef and remove from the heat. Add the mayonnaise, pickles, mustard, ketchup, and bell pepper in a blender and mix the mixture until smooth and well combined.

Now combine the lettuce, tomatoes, and cheddar cheese in a mixing bowl and add the ground beef and dressing until evenly coated.

Pan-Fried Pepperoni Pizzas

Ingredients

- Six large eggs
- Six tablespoons of grated Parmesan cheese
- Three tablespoons of psyllium powder
- One and ½ teaspoon of Italian herbs
- 3 tablespoons of olive oil
- Nine tablespoons low-carb tomato sauce
- 4 and 1/2 ounces of grated mozzarella
- One and ½ grams of chopped pepperoni
- Three tablespoons of freshly cut basil

Instructions

Take a blender and combine the eggs, parmesan cheese, and psyllium husk powder with the Italian herbs and a pinch of salt. Mix the mixture until smooth and well combined. It will take about 30 seconds and then let it rest for 5 minutes. Now heat one tablespoon of oil in a skillet over medium heat. Pour the batter on the pan and divide it in a circle. Cook until browned underneath. Now turn the crust over and brown on the other side too. Take a baking tray, cover it with a foil, and place the pizza crust on it. Repeat the process with the remaining batter. Now spread three tablespoons of low-carb tomato sauce over each crust. Top them with diced pepperoni and grated cheese, then roast until the cheese browns. Then sprinkle them with fresh basil. Then cut the pizza to serve.

Chicken Zoodle Alfredo

Ingredients

- 2 chicken fillets
- 1 tablespoon of olive oil
- Salt and pepper
- 2 tablespoons of butter
- ¼ cup of whipped cream
- ¼ cup of grated Parmesan cheese
- 200 grams of zucchini

Instructions

Heat the olive oil over medium heat. Add the chicken to the skillet and season with salt and pepper. Cook the chicken for 6 to 7 minutes per side and cut the chicken into strips. Now heat the skillet over medium heat and add the butter.

Add the cream and Parmesan cheese to the butter and cook them until they thicken. Now spiral the zucchini and then toss it in the sauce mix with the chicken. Then c ALSO there is about 2 minutes until the zucchini cooked. Serve hot.

Cabbage and sausage skillet

Ingredients

- Six large Italian sausage links
- ½ cup sliced green cabbage

- 2 tablespoons of butter
- ¼ cup of sour cream
- ¼ cup of mayonnaise
- Salt and pepper

Instructions

Take a skillet and cook the sausages over medium heat until evenly browned, then cut into slices. Now heat the skillet over medium heat and add the butter. Add the cabbage to the pan and cook for about 3 to 4 minutes until wilted. Then add the sliced sausage and sour cream together with the mayonnaise to the cabbage. Now season with salt and pepper and let it simmer for 10 minutes.

Gyro salad with avo-Tzatziki

Ingredients

- 1 tablespoon of olive oil
- 1 pound ground lamb
- ½ medium chopped yellow onion
- ¼ cup of chicken stock
- Four teaspoons of lemon juice
- ½ teaspoon of dried oregano
- ½ teaspoon of dried thyme
- ½ English cucumber
- 1 medium ripe avocado
- Two teaspoons freshly cut mint
- 1 teaspoon of freshly chopped dill
- 6 cups chopped romaine lettuce

Instructions

Heat the oil over medium heat in a large skillet, then add the lamb.
Cook the lamb for 3 minutes, stirring regularly, then add the onions. Continue to cook the lamb until well prepared, and the onion softens. Then add the chicken stock, two teaspoons of lemon juice, oregano, and thyme. Simmer for 5 minutes after seasoning with salt and pepper to taste. Now grate the cucumber. Spread them evenly on a clean towel and squeeze out the moisture. Now place the grated cucumber in a blender and add the avocado, two teaspoons lemon juice, mint, and the dill with a grain of salt as well. Mix

the mixture until smooth. Serve this freshly prepared gyro over the chopped lettuce and with a spoonful of avo-tzatziki.

WEEK 3

	Breakfast	Lunch	Supper	Total number of instructions
Sunday	3 Cloud Buns with three tablespoons. Peanut butter and - 3 slices of thick-cut bacon	Mozzarella Tuna melt	Cheesy Single-Serve Lasagna	Calories: 1605 Fat: 116.5g Protein: 114.5g Net Carbs: 28.5g
Monday	Bacon Breakfast Bombs	Sandwiches with avocado, eggs, and salami	Crispy Chipotle chicken thighs	Calories: 1,525 Fat: 118.5g Protein: 99.5g Net carbohydrates: 12 g
Tuesday	T RIE-Cheese Pizza frittata with- 3 Slices Thick-Cut Bacon	Leftover mozzarella tuna melt	Pepperoni, ham and cheddar Stromboli	Calories: 1,660 Fat: 121 g Protein: 119 g Net carbohydrates: 22.5 g
Wed.	3 Cloud Buns with three tablespoons. Peanut butter and - 2 slices of thick-cut bacon	Leftover T cheese Pizza Frittata with 2 slices of thick-cut bacon	Leftover Pepperoni, Ham and Cheddar Stromboli	Calories: 1,640 Fat: 130.5 g Protein: 100.5 g Net Carbs: 20.5 g
Thursday	Leftover Bacon Breakfast Bombs	Leftover sandwiches with	Leftover crispy Chipotle	Calories: 1,625 Fat: 126.5g

		avocado, eggs, and salami with 1 slice of thick-cut bacon	chicken thighs	Protein: 106.5g Net Carbs: 12.5g
Friday	Leftover Three-Cheese Pizza frittata with- 2 Slices of Thick-Cut Bacon	Leftover Pepperoni, Ham and Cheddar Stromboli	Spring salad with steak and sweet dressing	Calories: 1,585 Fat: 120.5g Protein: 108g Net carbohydrates: 13.5 g
Saturday	Leftover T cheese Pizza Frittata with 2 slices of thick-cut bacon	Mushroom soup with a fried egg and two slices of thick-cut bacon	Leftover spring salad with steak and sweet dressing	Calories: 1,665 Fat: 130.5g Protein: 110g Net Carbs: 13.5

Easy Cloud Buns

Ingredients

- 3 large eggs
- 1/8 teaspoon of tartar
- 3 ounces chopped cream cheese

Instructions

Preheat your oven to 300 ° F. Take a parchment paper and line it with a baking sheet. Now beat the egg whites until foamy and then add the tartar cream until it is shiny white and opaque with soft peaks. Take a separate bowl and beat in the cream cheese and egg yolks until well combined.

Fold the egg white mixture through the beaten material. Divide the batter between the ¼ cup baking trays and keep them 2 centimeters apart. Bake them for 30 minutes until the rolls are well baked and feel firm.

Bacon Breakfast Bombs

Ingredients

- 4 slices of thickly sliced bacon
- 2 large eggs
- ¼ cup diced butter
- 2 tablespoons of mayonnaise
- Salt and pepper

Instructions

First, take the bacon rashers and cook them in a large skillet over medium heat until crispy. Allow the bacon to cool slightly, chop finely and set it aside, keeping the bacon fat. Fill a saucepan with water, and a pinch of salt, then bring to a boil. Add the eggs and cook them for 10 minutes before putting them in an ice-water bath.

Let the eggs cool, peel and chop coarsely. Add the chopped eggs to the butter and mash them. Then add the mayonnaise, salt, pepper, and also. Stir in reserved bacon fat, cover mixture, and set aside for 30 minutes. Divide the egg mixture into six portions and roll them into balls and roll in the ground bacon. Serve hot and store the leftovers in the refrigerator. Servings: 3 bombs.

Three-cheese Pizza Frittata

Ingredients

- ½ bag of frozen spinach
- Six large eggs
- 2 tablespoons of olive oil
- ½ teaspoon of dried Italian herbs

- Salt and pepper
- ¼ cup of ricotta cheese
- ¼ cup of grated Parmesan cheese
- Two and ½ grams of grated mozzarella cheese
- 1 ounce sliced pepperoni

Instructions

Preheat your oven to 375 ° F. Take a pie plate and grease it with cooking spray. Thaw the frozen spinach and squeeze the water. Take a bowl and beat the eggs, olive oil, Italian herbs, salt, pepper, and in it. Then add the ricotta cheese, parmesan, and drained spinach until well combined.

Pour the prepared mixture on the pie plate and cover with mozzarella and pepperoni. Bake the pie for 35 to 40 minutes until the egg is firm and the cheese is lightly browned.

Mozzarella Tuna melt

Ingredients

- 1 tablespoon of olive oil
- ½ cup chopped yellow onion
- 8 ounces of canned tuna
- ¼ cup of mayonnaise
- 2 beaten large eggs
- 2 ounces of grated mozzarella cheese
- Salt and pepper
- One thinly sliced green onion

Instructions

Heat the olive oil in a frying pan. Now add the onions and cook until translucent for about 5 minutes. Drain the excess water from the tuna. Peel it in the pan and add the remaining ingredients. Season with salt and pepper and cook for 2 minutes or until the cheese has melted. Place it in a bowl and cover with sliced green onion to serve.

Sandwiches with avocado egg and salami

Ingredients

- 4 Easy Cloud Buns
- 1 teaspoon of butter
- Four large eggs
- 1 medium tomato and cut into 4 slices
- 1 ounce thinly sliced fresh mozzarella
- 1 thinly sliced small avocado
- 2 ounces of sliced salami
- Salt and pepper

Instructions

Take the cloud buns and roast them on a baking tray in the oven until golden brown. Now heat and melt the butter in a large skillet over medium heat. Divide the cracked eggs in the pan and season with salt and pepper. Cook the eggs until cooked to the desired level and place one on top of each cloud bun. Now serve the sandwiches with sliced tomato, mozzarella, avocado, and salami.

Mushroom soup with a fried egg

Ingredients

- 1 teaspoon of olive oil
- 4 thinly sliced white mushrooms
- 100 grams of cauliflower with rice
- 1 cup of vegetable stock
- 3 tablespoons of whipped cream
- 2 tablespoons of grated cheese
- 1 teaspoon of butter
- 1 large egg

Instructions

Take a small saucepan and heat the oil in it over medium heat. Then add the mushrooms and cook them for 6 minutes.

Add the cauliflower, vegetable stock, and whipped cream to the pan. Season with salt and pepper and add the cheese. Simmer the soup until the consistency matches the desired level, then remove from the heat. Fry the eggs in the butter and serve over the soup.

Cheesy Single-Serve Lasagna

Ingredients

* 3 tablespoons low-carb marinara sauce
* 1 small thinly sliced in zucchini circles
* 2 tablespoons of ricotta cheese
* 3 ounces of grated mozzarella
* Dried oregano

Instructions

Place 1 tablespoon of marinara sauce in a microwave-safe bowl. Take the zucchini slices and divide a third of them over the sauce and cover with a tablespoon of ricotta cheese. Now repeat the process and make the layers of sauce, zucchini, and ricotta.

Finally, top with the leftover zucchini and a tablespoon of marinara. Sprinkle the top with mozzarella, then microwave for 3 to 4 minutes until the mixture is heated well, and the cheese is melted. Sprinkle with dried oregano and serve warm.

Crispy Chipotle chicken thighs

Ingredients

* ½ teaspoon of chipotle chili powder
* ¼ teaspoon of garlic powder
* ¼ teaspoon of onion powder
* ¼ teaspoon of ground coriander
* ¼ teaspoon of smoked paprika
* 12 grams of boneless chicken thighs
* Salt and pepper
* 1 tablespoon of olive oil
* 3 cups of fresh baby spinach

Instructions

Take a small bowl and combine the chipotle chili powder, garlic powder, onion powder, cilantro, and smoked paprika. Flatten the chicken thigh by stamping on it and season with salt and pepper on both sides.

Now cut these chicken thighs in half. Heat the oil in a heavy skillet over medium heat. Now add the chicken thighs skin side down to the pan and sprinkle them with the spice mixture. Cook these chicken thighs on the first side for 8 minutes. Then turn over and bake for 3 to 5 minutes on the other side. Add the spinach to the pan and cook for 3 minutes until wilted. Serve them on a bed of wilted spinach.

Pepperoni, ham and cheddar Stromboli
Ingredients

- 1 and ¼ cups of grated mozzarella
- ¼ cup of almond flour
- 3 tablespoons of coconut flour
- 1 teaspoon of dried Italian herbs
- Salt and pepper
- 1 large beaten egg
- 6 ounces of sliced deli ham
- 2 ounces of sliced pepperoni
- 4 ounces of sliced cheddar cheese
- 1 tablespoon of melted butter
- 6 cups of fresh salad greens

Instructions

Preheat your oven to 400 ° F. Take a parchment paper and line it with baking sheet. Take the microwave-safe bowl and melt the mozzarella cheese in it until it can be stirred smooth.

Take a separate bowl and mix together the almond flour, coconut flour, and dried Italian herbs.

Now pour the melted cheese into the flour mixture and work this together with some salt and pepper. Add in the egg into the four and knead into a dough, then spread on a piece of parchment. Now place a piece of parchment on the money and roll the dough into an oval. Take a knife and cut diagonal slits along the edges, leaving the center 10 centimeters untouched. Spread the ham and cheese slices in the middle of the dough fold the strips on the top of the mixture. Brush the top of the money with butter. Bake for 15 to 20 minutes until the dough is browned. Cut and serve with a small salad.

Spring salad with steak and sweet dressing
Ingredients

- 2 slices of thick-cut bacon

- 2 tablespoons of white wine vinegar
- 2 tablespoons of olive oil
- 2 tablespoons of fresh raspberries
- Liquid stevia
- 4 cups of fresh spring vegetables
- 1 ounce of roasted pine nuts
- 1 tablespoon of butter
- 7 grams of beef steak

Instructions

Take a skillet and cook the bacon in it over medium heat until very crispy. Chop the bacon. Take a blender and combine the white wine vinegar, olive oil, raspberries, and liquid stevia. Mix the ingredients until smooth and well combined. After that, take a large bowl and mix in the spring greens, toasted pine nuts, and crumbled bacon. Sprinkle the dressing, and divide the salad between two plates. Now take a skillet and melt the butter in it over medium-high heat, then add the steak. Season the steak with salt and pepper, then sear on one side for about 3 to 4 minutes. Now turn the steak over and cook from the other side to the desired level. Let it rest for 5 minutes. After cutting, add the steak to the salad.

WHAT CHANGES OCCUR IN YOUR BODY DURING THE KETO DIET?

Many people today run to the idea of a low-carb diet. They do not consult their doctor about this and start a ketogenic diet themselves, which is not the right way at all. In the course of losing weight, they forget the precaution and get the results they never expected. The ketogenic diet does much better and worse for your body than just losing weight. The following changes occur in your body when you are on a keto diet.

Rapid weight loss

One of the promising things at a keto diet is that the person loses weight quickly. A keto specialist says a keto diet has an infamous reputation for rapid and aggressive fat loss. Because the majority of the quick weight loss stories come from people with a very low-calorie diet and a low-fat diet. This does not happen with the ketogenic diet. It is not a starvation diet. It is the opposite of starvation diets. A keto diet should keep as many calories as possible, and it is highly recommended that your body should have the required calorie level depending on your weight. However, there is one thing about the keto diet that it is primarily a water diet. Initially, weight loss is fast, but when weight loss stops, people lose confidence in this diet and abandon it.

Keto flu

One of the most feared things about a ketogenic diet is the keto flu. By removing carbohydrates from your diet during the first days of the ketogenic diet, your body may experience some symptoms, including irritability, fatigue, headaches, mood swings, and insomnia. These are the symptoms of keto flu, which can be experienced when starting a ketogenic diet. The body can also experience brain fog, which results from changing energy sources in your diet, such as incorporating calories from carbohydrates into fats.

There is nothing to worry about these issues because they can be easily identified by eating more salt, potassium, and drinking more water.

Possibility of muscle cramps

It is possible that during the ketogenic diet, your body may experience muscle cramps. This is not due to your daily workouts, but the keto diet. Due to the lack of sodium and potassium in the body, these muscle cramps occur and can be easily treated by including more sodium and potassium in your diet. The professionals also highly recommend it. Because when a person starts a ketogenic diet, the sodium is removed from the liver and the body doesn't have enough resources to make up for this loss.

Improves insulin sensitivity

During your ketogenic diet, you don't consume foods containing sugar starch and carbohydrates, so it becomes a reason your body slowly raises blood sugar. This means that those people have better insulin sensitivity. It is best for people with type 2 diabetes blood.

Stinking breath

One thing that also happens to your body during a ketogenic diet is the stinky breath. It occurs when your body starts to burn carbohydrates, store them in the liver as glycogen, and then use it for energy purposes. Then it flashes the fats. This process creates ketones, the energy packs, and the process is called ketosis. When your body goes through the process of ketosis, it produces a large amount of acetone, causing your breath to smell. Many people also consider it a good sign that their body has started to burn fats.

The energy level increases

When your body enters the phase of ketosis and adapts to the ketogenic diet, your body's energy level begins to stabilize.
It is because of the reason that your body is going to burn fats for energy and also because you are removing the starchy and sugary elements from your diet and then start eating whole foods, which is your body's essential requirement. It is unlike other diets that increase energy levels; instead, it stabilizes.

Reduces inflammation

The leading cause of many diseases, especially heart disease, bowel disease, and cancer, is chronic inflammation. A ketogenic diet helps lower the levels of inflammation in your body and improves arthritis, eczema, protects the brain, and many other diseases.

Ability to develop a rash on your body

Another side effect of the ketogenic diet is keto rash. It happens due to vitamin deficiency in the body during the ketogenic diet. It can appear as raised red skin with a brown or light pink color. While the keto rash is not severe and dangerous, it can be irritating and itchy. When you experience this keto rash, just increase the diet you are on and take multivitamins, and it will be better. And if the situation is still not cured, you should consult the doctor.

Change in urine

Frequent urination is another side effect of a ketogenic diet. The color and smell of urine are also different. It may be because ketones are excreted with other products and retain more water than the daily routine.

Stomach problems

Diarrhea and constipation are the two stomachs and digestion problems people have a ketogenic diet face. It is due to the reduction of carbohydrates from your diet.
This can be cured by taking more green and non-starchy vegetables like avocado, kale, or broccoli.

Effects of irregularity during a keto diet

The following are some reasons and their effects that occur when you are not regularly on the ketogenic diet:
Drinking too little water during a ketogenic diet does not help reduce weight. It is always recommended to take more fluids and drink more water during a ketogenic diet.
Dairy products are an ingredient of a keto diet because they are low in carbohydrates and high in fats. However, an excessive intake of milk fats can lead to irregularities and overeating. So always be moderate with eating these products.
More often, it is a fact that people think in this way that fats are directly proportional to gaining weight. And during the keto diet, they take in fewer fats than recommended. This can be dangerous to the metabolism and

function of hormones in your body. Since you cut carbohydrates from your diet, you should also take the right fats.

During the keto diet, you don't crave snacks because it has a satisfying element of its own. But you can only use the snacks in moderation if you are too hungry between meals. It is not appropriate to take too many snacks because they can easily increase calories.

During a ketogenic diet, it is recommended that people sleep peacefully for 7-8 hours. If they don't get this amount of sleep, then they will crave sugary foods, and increase their sickness stress levels. It will only result in you getting extra fats.

KETO DIET RECIPES

If you are keto, you recognize that there are enough no-nos in classic raincoat & cheese. This version eliminates all difficulty levels for children without sacrificing taste. The pork rind topping is completely optional. We predict it adds a pleasant crunch.

INGREDIENTS:
FOR the raincoat & CHEESE

- Butter, for baking dish
- 2 medium cauliflowers, cut roses
- 2 tablespoons. extra virgin oil
- Kosher salt
- 1 c. cream
- 6 oz. cheese, cubes
- 4 c. sliced cheese
- 2 c. sliced cheese
- 1 tbsp. sauce (optional)
- Freshly ground black pepper

FOR THE TOPPING

- 4 Oz. pork rind, crushed
- 1/4 c. freshly grated Parmesan cheese
- 1 tbsp. extra virgin oil
- 2 tablespoons. freshly cut parsley, for garnish

DIRECTIONS
Preheat the kitchen appliance to 375 ° and butter a 9 "-x-13" baking dish. During a huge bowl, toss cauliflower with a few tablespoons of oil and season with salt. Unfold cauliflower on two huge baking sheets and fry until tender and golden brown, about forty minutes.

Meanwhile, heat the cream in a huge pan over medium heat. Talk about simmering, then reduce heat to low and stir in cheese until melted. Remove from the heat, add sauce if you wish to use it and season with salt and pepper, then stir in the roasted cauliflower. Style and season extra if necessary.

Transfer the mixture to the baking tin. In a medium bowl, stir to mix pork rinds, parmesan, and oil. Sprinkle the mixture in an excellent layer over cauliflower and cheese.

Bake until golden brown, 15 minutes. If desired, turn the kitchen appliance over so that it can roast for a few minutes.

Garnish with parsley before serving.

Keto cooked chicken

To make a Keto-friendly cooked chicken, we tended to skip the flour and went for pork rind and Parmesan. Almond flour helps to stick to everything in addition to a beautifully sharp chicken. We tend to fry this chicken together to skip any excess oil; however, it still bakes in a deformity that you would just swear was cooked. Also like to use thighs or drumsticks, just keep in mind that the baking time is longer!

INGREDIENTS

FOR THE CHICKEN

- 6 chicken breast with bones and skin (about 4 lbs.)
- Kosher salt
- Freshly ground black pepper
- 2 huge eggs
- 1/2 c. cream
- 3/4 c. almond flour
- 1 1/2 c. finely ground pork rind
- 1/2 c. freshly grated Parmesan cheese
- 1 teaspoon. garlic powder
- 1/2 tsp. paprika

FOR THE Spicy salad dressing

- 1/2 c. mayonnaise
- 1 1/2 tsp. hot sauce

DIRECTIONS

Heat kitchen appliance s to 400 ° and conduit outsize baking plates dry with towels with a baking paper and pat the chicken, salt, and pepper is also on. Beat in a small bowl along with eggs and cream. In another shallow bowl, mix the rest of the things and make a mixture. Start one by one by dipping the chicken into the mixture and squeezing it into the almond flour mixture to coat. Place the chicken on a prepared baking sheet.

Bake until chicken is golden brown and the internal temperature reaches 165 °, with respect to forty - five minutes.

Meanwhile, make the dipping sauce: In a medium bowl, mix dressing and sauce. Add extra sauce bets at the most loved spiciness level.

Serve chicken heat with dipping sauce.

Broccoli dish

Broccoli dish is an excellent meal preparation formula. In addition to being extensive and healthy, we expect it to be an even higher consistency day. If you're a feeder, swap the bacon for a diced avocado - the thickness can be a nice compliment to the spicy broccoli.

INGREDIENTS

- In court
- kosher salt
- 3 cups of broccoli, bite-size items
- 1/2 c. chopped cheese
- 1/4 purple onion, thinly sliced
- 1/4 c. cooked sliced almonds
- 3 slices of bacon, medium and broken
- 2 tablespoons. freshly cut chives

FOR THE DRESSING

- 2/3 c. mayonnaise
- 3 tbsp. apple acetum
- 1 tbsp. mustard
- Kosher salt
- Freshly ground black pepper

DIRECTIONS

In a medium saucepan or pan, bring half a dozen cups of preserved water to a boil. While looking forward to the water for cooking, prepare an oversized bowl of drinking water.

Add broccoli florets to the boiling water and cook until tender, one to a few minutes. Take it away with a slotted spoon and place it in the ready-to-drink water bowl. Let the florets cool during a sieve.

In a medium bowl, beat the ingredients for the dressing—season with salt and pepper.

Combine all the dish ingredients in a huge bowl and pour overdressing. Toss until the ingredients are combined and covered with a dressing. Cool until ready to serve.

Keto cheesecake

A breeze to cook makes this the right evening dinner for everyone and will make you spend a lot of time with a Keto cheesecake for dessert!

INGREDIENTS

FOR THE MEATBALLS

- 1 pound burger
- 1 garlic clove, minced
- 1/2 c. chopped cheese
- 1/4 c. freshly grated parmesan cheese and plenty for serving
- 2 tablespoons. freshly cut parsley
- 1 huge egg, beaten
- 1 teaspoon. kosher salt
- 1/2 tsp. freshly ground black pepper
- 2 tablespoons. extra virgin vegetable oil

FOR THE SAUCE

- 1 medium onion, finely chopped
- 2 cloves of garlic, minced
- 1 (28-oz.) Will crush tomatoes
- 1 teaspoon. dried oregano
- Kosher salt
- Freshly ground black pepper

DIRECTIONS

In a huge bowl, mix beef, garlic, mozzarella, Parmesan cheese, parsley, egg, salt, and pepper. Type in sixteen meatballs.

Fry the oil in a large saucepan over medium heat, then add meatballs and cook, often turning, golden brown on all sides, about ten minutes. Remove from the pan and place on a paper towel-lined plate.

Add to a constant pan of onion and cook until soft, 5 minutes. Add garlic and cook until sweet, one minute a lot. Add sauces and tomatoes and later add meatballs back to the pan, cap, and simmer until the sauce has thickened, 15 minutes. Garnish with Parmesan cheese before serving.

Cheesy Bacon Ranch Chicken

If you're trying a keto diet, these stray chicken breasts will build the right quick and easy evening dinner. The ranch seasoning is elective, but wouldn't you?

INGREDIENTS

- 4 slices of thickly sliced bacon
- 4 boneless chicken breasts (about 1 3/4 lbs.)
- Kosher salt
- Freshly ground black pepper
- 2 teaspoons of ranch seasoning
- 1 1/2 c. chopped cheese
- Chopped chives, for garnish

DIRECTIONS

In a huge saucepan over medium heat, cook the bacon, turning once, until soft, about eight minutes.

Transfer to a paper towel-lined plate. Pour almost a few tablespoons of bacon fat from the pan. Season the chicken with salt and pepper. Put the pan back on medium heat, add chicken and cook until golden brown and just mediocre, about a half dozen minutes per side.

Reduce heat to low and sprinkle chicken with ranch herbs and primer with cheese. Fry the pan and cook until the cheese is meltable and sparkling about five minutes.

Crumble and sprinkle bacon and baskets before serving on prime. Keto Bacon Sushi

Keto snacks

Eating a keto diet means you have fewer choices for snacking. No fear! These very little boys can satisfy all your cravings for snacks: they are salty, creamy, and crunchy; however, they will not be easy to carry around. We tend to go for carrots, cucumbers, and avocado for our stuffing; however, the choices are endless. Turn it on with paprika, celery, radish, or whatever else you have on hand!

INGREDIENTS

- 6 slices of bacon, cut in half
- 2 Persian cucumbers, thinly sliced
- 2 medium carrots, thinly sliced
- 1 avocado, sliced
- 4 Oz. cheese softens
- Sesame seeds, for garnish

DIRECTIONS

Heat kitchen appliance s to 400°.line the sheet with aluminum foil also work with a cooling rack. Layer the bacon halves well and cook until crispy, but still smooth, eleven to thirteen minutes. Meanwhile, cut cucumbers, carrots, and avocado into pieces about the width of the bacon. When the bacon is cool enough to touch, fold a good layer of cheese onto each slice.

Spread the vegetables evenly over the bacon and place them on one finish. Roll vegetables up tightly. Garnish with benne seeds and serve.

Keto Taco Oven Dish

It's super easy, extraordinarily sturdy, and it has a touch of the jalapeño. Clean with our keto frosty for a decadent and delicious keto party!

INGREDIENTS

- 1 tbsp. extra virgin vegetable oil
- 1/2 yellow onion, diced
- 2 pounds of beef
- 2 tablespoons. kosher salt
- Freshly ground black pepper
- 2 tablespoons. combine keto taco spices
- 1 jalapeño, without seeds and chopped, and extra cut as a garnish
- 6 giant eggs, gently crushed
- 2 c. sliced Mexican cheese
- 2 tablespoons. freshly cut parsley leaves
- 1 c. sour cream, for serving (optional)

DIRECTIONS

Heat the cooking apparatus is up to 350°. Heat oil in an extra-large pan over medium heat. Add onions and cook until soft in 2 minutes.

Add beef and season with salt and pepper. Cook, breaking the meat with a picket spoon, so far not pink, 6 minutes. Sprinkle with taco seasoning and jalapeño and cook, stirring, until the herbs are gently cooked, 1 minute. Drain and allow to cool slightly.

In a giant bowl, beat eggs and add the meat mixture. Unfold the mixture into a protruding layer on the bottom of a 2-quart baking dish. Sprinkle with cheese.

Bake until set, covering twenty - five minutes.

Sprinkle with parsley and fill each slice with a small indeterminate amount of cream and jalapeño, if desired.

Chicken keto parmesan

INGREDIENTS

- 4 boneless chicken breasts
- Kosher salt
- Freshly ground black pepper
- 1 c. almond flour
- 3 giant eggs, beaten
- 3 c. freshly grated cheese, and plenty for serving
- 2 teaspoons of garlic powder
- 1 teaspoon. onion powder
- 2 teaspoons of dried oregano
- Vegetable oil
- 3/4 c. low-carb, sugar-free pasta sauce
- 1 1/2 c. sliced cheese
- Fresh basil leaves, as a topping

DIRECTIONS

Heat the cooking apparatus is up to 400 °. Cut the chicken fillets crosswise in 0.5 with a sharp knife. Season the chicken on both sides with salt and pepper.

Place eggs and almond flour in a few separate shallow bowls. In an unusually third shallow bowl, mix cheese, garlic powder, onion powder, and oregano— season with salt and pepper. Working one by one, dip chicken cutlets in almond flour, then egg and then cheese mixture, press to coat.

In a large skillet over medium heat, heat a few tablespoons of oil. Add chicken and cook until golden brown and stewed for a few to three minutes per facet. Add batches if necessary, and add plenty of oil if necessary. Transfer cooked cutlets to a 9 "- x-13" baking dish, unfold the pasta sauce on each scallop, and high with cheese. Bake until cheese is floury, ten to twelve minutes. If desired, toast until the cheese is golden brown, 3 minutes.

Top with basil and plenty of cheese before serving.

FREQUENTLY ASKED QUESTIONS ABOUT KETO DIET

What is the ketosis process in a ketogenic diet?

During a ketogenic diet, when your body undergoes the process of breaking down fats and carbohydrates for energy extraction or storing those broken fat fuel in the form of ketones, it is called the process of ketosis.

Is a ketogenic diet safe or not?

The ketogenic diet is perfectly healthy and also a safe diet compared to other diets. Before starting a keto diet, and it is strongly recommended to consult a doctor. You should also be extra careful in the following situations:

- If you have a heart condition.
- Especially if you have diabetes type 1.
- If you are breastfeeding.

What kind of food should be consumed during a ketogenic diet?

A simple guide to foods to eat during a ketogenic diet is to eat low carb and high fat.

Is a ketogenic diet safe for our kidneys?

A ketogenic diet is completely safe for your kidneys. Many people ask this question because they confuse fats with proteins.
Excess protein is harmful to your kidneys, while a ketogenic diet is high in fats.

Which drinks are suitable during the Keto Diet?

It is recommended to drink too much water if you want to drink coffee or tea, then without sugar, and you can also drink a glass of wine, but only occasionally.

CONCLUSION

The low carbohydrate approach is recommended by doctors to patients that has saved many lives. Some experienced physicians believe that a ketogenic diet may be a type of drug, and this drug really works between doctors and patients. By following the ketogenic diet, you can hardly become obsessed with doctors. This ensures that you are ready enough to try things for yourself with little or no point in the direction of the doctor. On a daily basis, you feel like making a difference in your life. Today, it is quite common to examine doctors who have a low-carbohydrate mode in their patients. The recommendation of the doctor for a ketogenic diet shows the great desire and the importance of a ketogenic diet for a healthy life.